IMPROVING YOUR MENTAL GAME:

A Sports Psychiatry Pocket Guide

for Athletes, Coaches, & Athletic Trainers

Pamela Smith, MD

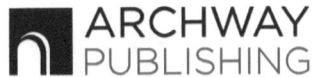

ARCHWAY
PUBLISHING

Archway Publishing books may be ordered
through booksellers or by contacting:

Archway Publishing
1663 Liberty Drive
Bloomington, IN 47403
www.archwaypublishing.com
1 (888) 242-5904

Because of the dynamic nature of the Internet, any web addresses or
links contained in this book may have changed since publication and
may no longer be valid. The views expressed in this work are solely those
of the author and do not necessarily reflect the views of the publisher,
and the publisher hereby disclaims any responsibility for them.

Any people depicted in stock imagery provided by Shutterstock are
models, and such images are being used for illustrative purposes only.
Certain stock imagery © Shutterstock.

ISBN: 978-1-4808-4414-8 (sc)
ISBN: 978-1-4808-4415-5 (e)

Library of Congress Control Number: 2017902800

Print information available on the last page.

Archway Publishing rev. date: 03/08/2017

ABOUT THE AUTHOR

Pamela Smith, MD completed specialty training in psychiatry at New York–Presbyterian University Hospital of Columbia & Cornell and later served on the faculty of the UCLA Medical School, the staff of the UCLA Neuropsychiatric Hospital (NPH), and the visiting faculty of the UCLA Department of Psychology. Her training has included externships with sports medicine practitioners providing clinical interventions and developing mental skills training programs for amateur and professional athletes and performing artists. While at UCLA/NPH, she served as the Medical Director of the Partial Hospital & Intensive Outpatient Programs and attending psychiatrist for varied services (inpatient, outpatient, emergency room, & consultation-liaison).

Dr. Smith has also worked in developing countries as a mental health consultant on humanitarian aid projects in collaboration with nonprofit organizations and agencies including the International Medical Corps (IMC), World Health Organization (WHO), UNICEF, and UNHCR. As a mental health consultant, she trained clinicians to provide basic mental health interventions in settings where mental health resources were limited and created community sporting activities for youth as a means for psychosocial support and development.

ACKNOWLEDGEMENTS

A special thanks to Aleksandra Bajic-Lucas, PharmD for assistance with the chapter, "Overview of Banned Substances." Much gratitude is extended to Whitney A. Relf, MA, PhD (Disabilities Consultant) for review of the section, "Athletes with Disabilities" and to Ashley Relf, MA (Performance Coach) for contributions to the section, "Mental Wellness, Balance, & Life Skills."

TABLE OF CONTENTS

I. INTRODUCTION

Sports psychiatry uses psychological, neuroscientific, and medical knowledge to address optimal performance and well-being of athletes. The "mental game" refers not only to a mind that has been conditioned through mental skills training for optimal performance, but also to a broader *mindset* that includes an awareness of psychosocial issues and mental conditions that potentially impact optimal performance.

This pocket guide is a practical, concise, and convenient booklet for college and professional athletes, coaches, and athletic trainers with topics including:

1) Core psychological techniques for improving athletic performance (e.g. imagery, goal setting, self-talk, relaxation).

2) Tips and exercises for managing focus, negative self-talk, pressure, daily learning & growth, commitment, self-defeating distractions, fear, motivation, riding the bench, taking responsibility, controlling emotions, self-belief & confidence, trust & consistency, and pregame warm-up.

3) Psychosocial issues impacting performance (e.g. team cohesion, managing team conflict, coping with injury, end of career issues).

4) Mental conditions associated with the competitive sports environment (e.g. anxiety,

depression, substance abuse, concussion, eating disorders).

In addition, information on banned substances (of which many are psychoactive), athletes with disabilities, and brain health maintenance (e.g. sleep and nutrition for optimal brain & neuromuscular function) is included.

II. MENTAL SKILLS TRAINING (MST)

Mental skills have been defined as a set of trainable mental abilities that are at the basis of successful learning and performance. Mental or psychological skills include confidence, motivation, attention or focus, arousal/anxiety control, and general self-awareness. These skills may be developed or improved using varied methods or tools including relaxation (e.g. breathing & progressive muscle relaxation), self-talk, imagery, and goal-setting. In this section, the application of each of these core tools is outlined.

1) TOOLS

A) Relaxation: Breathing & Progressive Muscle Relaxation

<u>Breathing</u>

Deep Breathing

Deep or diaphragmatic breathing to reduce anxiety or stress involves taking in (through the nose) a slow, large deep breath (using the diaphragm muscle), holding it briefly, and slowly exhaling (through the mouth). This type of breathing is associated with decreased heart rate, reduced blood pressure, and stimulation of the parasympathetic nervous system which plays a role in calming the body. It is used often for arousal/anxiety control, and to refocus (for example, after mistakes). A variety of techniques have been described for effective deep breathing - one example is provided on the following page.

Deep Breathing Exercise:

- Take a slow, deep breath in through the **nose** (to the count of 4). Be sure to inhale deeply using the diaphragm instead of chest (visualize a balloon filling with air).
- Hold it briefly.
- Slowly exhale (over 8 seconds) through the **mouth** (visualize a balloon losing its air).
- Do this exercise several times daily to get it ingrained in your mind, then incorporate it into your warm-up before practice or before a game (e.g. 5x/day including when you wake up; before breakfast, lunch, & dinner; and at bedtime).

Fast Breathing

Fast or shallow breathing involves pushing out, in quick succession, breaths from the throat and chest (as in panting). This type of breathing is associated with increasing the heart rate, increasing blood pressure, and stimulating the sympathetic nervous system which has an "energizing" effect on the body. This type of breathing is used in moments when energy is low and one needs to get "psyched-up."

Fast Breathing Exercise:

Open your mouth and push out 5 quick, shallow, "panting-like" breaths (push air from the throat and upper chest instead of from the abdomen or diaphragm). At the same time, visualize an image of someone or something that can be energizing to you (e.g. an engine revving up).

- Allow 2 seconds to pass then repeat, pushing 5 quick breaths through your **_nose_**.
- Repeat 4 cycles, alternating between fast breathing through the mouth and through the nose.
- Do this exercise several times daily to get it ingrained in your mind, then incorporate it into your warm-up prior to practice or a game (e.g. 5x/day including when you wake up; before breakfast, lunch, & dinner; and at bedtime).

<u>Progressive Muscle Relaxation</u>—Used for sleep; recovery after activity; to reduce pain/optimize healing.

Exercise:

For each of the muscle groups in your body, tense the muscles for 5–10 seconds, then relax for 10 seconds. Only tense your muscles moderately (not to the point of inducing pain). Don't force the release of the muscle tension - simply let go of the tension in your muscles and allow them to become relaxed. Relax your muscles in the following order:

Hands — clench one fist tightly, then relax. Do the same with the other hand.

Lower arms — bend your hand down at the wrist, as though you were trying to touch the underside of your arm, then relax.

Upper arms — bend your elbows and tense your arms. Feel the tension in your upper arm, then relax.

Shoulders — lift your shoulders up as if trying to touch your ears with them, then relax.

Neck — stretch your neck gently to the left, then forward, then to the right, then to the back in a slow rolling motion, then relax.

Forehead and scalp — raise your eyebrows, then relax.

Eyes — look about, rotating your eyes, then relax.

Jaw — clench your teeth (just to tighten the muscles), then relax.

Tongue — press your tongue against the roof of your mouth, then relax.

Chest — breathe in deeply to inflate your lungs, then breath out and relax.

Stomach — suck your tummy in to tighten the muscle,

then relax.

Upper back — pull your shoulders forward with your arms at your side, then relax.

Lower back — while sitting, lean your head and upper back forward, rolling your back into a smooth arc thus tensing the lower back, then relax.

Buttocks — tighten your buttocks, then relax.

Thighs — while sitting, push your feet firmly into the floor, then relax.

Calves — lift your toes off the ground towards your shins, then relax.

Feet — gently curl your toes down so that they are pressing into the floor, then relax.

B) Self-talk

Definition & Science Behind Self-Talk

In general, self-talk is defined as the act or practice of talking to oneself either silently or aloud. In sport, self-talk has been defined as external and internal dialogues applied to offer instruction and/or reinforcement to one's performance. Self-talk has been a tool used by athletes to improve or enhance mental skills important for performance including focus, arousal regulation ('psyching-up" or "psyching-down"), and confidence.

The science behind self-talk suggests that, through possible brain "remodeling" or reshaping of the brain physiology related to perception, self-talk may affect how you view yourself and therefore impact your feelings and behaviors. In simplistic terms, talking to oneself can set off of physiological process in the brain that can affect behavior.   In addition, verbalizing or speaking aloud one's self-talk may play a role in further reinforcing its effect.

Instructional vs Motivational Self-Talk

Self-talk may be instructional or motivational. Instructional self-talk involves talking yourself through a task with step-by-step reminders at each phase of the task. For example, instructional self-talk for a marksman may be: "Step 1, see the target; Step 2, straighten elbows, Step 3 lock onto the target, and Step 4 shoot..."

Motivational self-talk is used not only to bolster confidence, but also to decrease the anxiety and loss of focus that often accompanies decreased confidence. Examples of self-talk for confidence or motivation include "I can do this" or "Let's go!" Self-talk such as "breathe" or "I'm fine" can help decrease anxiety and tension. Repeating a word such as "focus" can help one get back on track and concentrate on the task at hand.

Negative vs Positive Self-Talk

Negative self-talk has been associated with diminishing performance on physical tasks and positive self-talk has been correlated with increased or positive performance. Strategies for managing negative self-talk include thought stopping & thought replacement; reframing; countering; and the use of positive self-affirming statements.

EXERCISE: Negative Thought-Stopping & Thought Replacement

A negative attitude and negative thinking are factors interfering with successful athletic performance. It is important to be able to have awareness of negative thoughts, find a way to stop them, and replace them with task-relevant, positive thoughts.

To stop negative thoughts:
1. Choose a "stop" command (e.g. visualize a stop sign; say the word, "STOP;" hear a bell); this will be used as a trigger to shift from negative to positive thinking.
2. Predict situations that can cause you to get negative (e.g. ref who missed the call; missed field goal; strikeout; foul called on you; missed free throw; unwarranted yellow card; didn't stick the landing, etc...).
3. Practice using the STOP command.
4. As you practice the STOP command, pair it with a physical gesture [e.g. turning away from the court or field, then staring into and seeing a **stop sign** in your racquet or mit (or on the field or floor)]. This helps to reinforce the command.
5. CONTINUOUSLY PRACTICE THE "STOP" COMMAND.

EXERCISE: Negative Thought-Stopping & Thought Replacement (continued)

After successfully stopping negative thoughts, it is important to replace them with positive, constructive thoughts. In addition to being positive, replacement thoughts should be short, specific, supportive, realistic, and expressed in 2nd person (i.e. use "you" instead of "I"). In selecting thoughts, use as a guideline positive thoughts a friend, coach, or teammate might say to encourage you. Examples are provided below.

Examples of positive replacement thoughts:

"Just go for it."

"This is tough, but you can do it…"

"Just keep trying…"

"You've done it before, you can do it again…"

"Don't quit, give it your best effort…"

"Everyone has a tough time, just hang in there…"

"Focus on what you can control…"

"Focus on your form, not your outcome…"

"Stay in the moment…"

"You hate this drill but you know it will make you better…"

"Let's go…"

"Right now…"

"Keep it going…"

"C'mon!"

Reframing

Reframing involves creating an alternative frame of reference, that is, looking at a situation or event from a different perspective. This is an important exercise for athletes because it teaches them to see failures as learning opportunities and to extract positives from negative experiences. The ability to reframe situations will allow athletes to maintain a positive and optimistic attitude even during hard times.

EXERCISE:

The first step to changing negative thoughts is to start taking particular notice of the themes and emotional tone of your thoughts. Listen to your internal comments; challenge those comments that are negative, defeatist or abusive; and deliberately reframe the thoughts so that they are positive, supportive and encouraging.

21

Example 1: "I've never done something as big as starting at quarterback before. What if I can't do it?"
Reframe: "I love a challenge. This assignment is simply a bigger version of my past success at the quarterback position. Time to step up."

Example 2: "I've fumbled the ball and now I'm going to lose the game for the team."
Reframe: "It's only the first quarter and there's plenty of game left. I've come back from mistakes in the past and can do it again today."

Countering

Countering involves creating an internal dialogue that uses facts, reason, and realistic functional explanations to refute the underlying false beliefs and assumptions that lead to negative thinking. For example, a player feels like he is not getting the opportunity to get into the game and is quick to believe, "the coach doesn't like me." This negative, unfounded belief can be countered with a more optimistic, realistic, and functional thought such as, "it's not that the coach doesn't like me...perhaps the coach wants to see more work from me or wants me to have more game-time experience before putting me in."

Positive Self-Affirming Statements

Self-affirming statements are short, positive, empowering phrases that are meant to be motivating and helpful in reminding the athlete of his or her strengths. To make them work, positive affirmations should be:

- Rehearsed regularly.
- Phrased positively.
- Framed in the present.
- Used in the first person — "I" statements.
- Focused on self-improvement, rather than compared to others.

- Descriptive, action words that generate emotion and feeling.
- Accurate, realistic and achievable.
- Aimed at developing personal traits (e.g. concentration, self-control, patience, etc).
- Focused on eliciting specific behaviors (e.g. "I manage my time efficiently and effectively now;" "I'm fit and healthy and I really enjoy practice on a daily basis;" "By setting regular goals and following through, I am becoming a more confident athlete").

<u>Summary: Effective Self-Talk</u>

In general, for self-talk to be effective, it should be:

1) Supportive but realistic.
2) Expressed positively rather than negatively (e.g. saying to self, "stay calm" instead of "don't get upset").
3) Focused on what you should do rather than on what you should avoid (say to yourself, "go for your shot" instead of "try not to get aced by my opponents shot").
4) Expressed in 2nd person. Use "you" rather than "I" when talking to yourself. When you think of yourself in second person, it allows you to give yourself more objective and useful feedback. For example, saying something like "Not bad, but you need to focus harder next time," is considered more motivating than "I wasn't focused enough" (which is a more self-defeating statement). Note: The exception to expressing self-talk in 2nd person is if you are using self-affirming statements which are usually expressed in 1st person.

C) Imagery (Visualization)

In sports, imagery (also referred to as visualization, mental training, and mental rehearsal) involves using all of your senses (not only sight, but also hearing, touch, smell, and even taste) to create or recreate an experience in your mind which aids you in developing or improving athletic skills and performance.

Research on imagery (motor imagery) tells us that the same neurological networks are used both to imagine movement and to actually move. In addition, imaging a movement over and over can have the same effect on the brain as physically practicing it repeatedly (and can actually lead to improving the movement as well). For example, if an athlete mentally images practicing her swing with a softball bat, the same brain networks that get stimulated when she swings an actual bat get activated. Additionally, if she continues to practice the swing in her mind repeatedly, when she practices again with the real bat, the swing may be improved. This has been the basis for using imagery as a tool for improving performance in athletics.

Imagery can be used to:

- Improve concentration.

- Build confidence.

- Control emotional responses.

- Acquire and practice sport skills.

- Acquire and practice strategy.

- Cope with pain and adversity.

- Solve problems.

Process of Imagery

The process of imagery involves:

1) Re-experiencing, in your mind, a best performance where skills were optimally executed or confidence, focus, or motivation were especially high.

2) Experiencing in detail not only the visual image of that performance but also the sounds, physical sensations, and even smells and tastes associated with the performance. The more associations that can be made, the stronger the imagery that can be used to improve your mental skills.

3) Scripts are often used to outline all details that are to be a part of the athlete's mental scenario.

Example 1: Using imagery to improve execution of a specific skill such as making perfect contact with the baseball (ideally resulting in a hit):

- While standing in the batter's box and practicing your swing, visualize a moment when you made perfect contact with the ball resulting in a positive outcome such as a hit or home run. NOTE: When using imagery to improve a skill or technique, focus on the *execution of the skill* instead of the end result or outcome. So, focus more on executing the proper hitting mechanics instead of hitting the home run. If you execute the skill properly the positive outcome will follow.

- Visual images: e.g. visualize the point on the field where you'd like to hit the ball (gap between the left & center fielders); visualize yourself in the proper stance that will allow you to hit it to that spot; visualize the sight of the ball coming toward the plate and making solid contact with the ball; and visualize the sight of the ball flying off the bat and landing at your point.

- Feelings or physical sensations in that moment: e.g. feel the wood bat in your relaxed, perfectly-positioned hands; feel the physical sensation of your legs, hips, arms, shoulders, and head in the optimal hitting position; and then feel yourself moving through the motion of the perfect swing.

- Sounds: e.g. hear the sound of the bat cracking the ball.

- Other sensations: associating other sensations present in the moment such as smell (e.g. fresh-cut grass on the field) and taste (e.g. cherry-flavored gum in your mouth) can further strengthen the imagery.

- Practice the visualization exercise repeatedly to reinforce the experience.

- If available, use photos or video to help reinforce the experience.

D) Goal-setting

Goal-setting improves performance by directing attention or focus; increasing effort and persistence; motivating one to learn new learning strategies; and increasing positive attitude.

Elements of Effective Goal-Setting:
- Make goals very specific, measurable, and observable.

- Clearly identify a time frame for attaining goals.

- Make goals of moderate difficulty level (not too easy or hard).

- Write goals down and monitor the progress (keep a journal).

- Use a mix of goals (i.e. a performance goal such as scoring 20 points in a basketball game and a process goal such as bending wrist and following through as you shoot the ball).

- Break down a long –term goal into a series of smaller goals (i.e. "baby steps").

- Set practice as well as competition goals.

- Share goals – helps you stay committed/others can hold you accountable.

Example: Goal-Setting

Long-term goal: *Increase my free throw shooting percentage to 65% from now (summer break) to when the school starts in the fall.*

Break down the long-term goal into specific short-term goals ("baby steps") and the strategies or actions to attain these goals. Short-term goals need to be realistic, attainable (no more than 3 goals), and expressed in a positive way:

Short-term goals (specific, measurable goals; no more than 3 goals)	Specific strategies, techniques, or actions to achieve the goal
1. Increase practice time	Stay an extra 30min after regular practice to practice free throws
2. Reassess my shot	Review video of the proper technique for shooting free throws and incorporate it into my shot
3. Develop a pre-shot routine	Before a shot: 1. use deep breathing to relax and self-talk to stay positive. 2. Visualize proper technique from video I studied. 3. Physically practice the proper technique with the ball in my hand but without actually shooting

Exercise: Setting Your Own Goals

Step 1: Determine a Long-term Goal

Long-term goal to achieve:

_____

Time-Frame you'd like to achieve goal in:

_____

Step 2: Break down the long-term goal into specific short-term "baby steps" goals and the strategies or actions to attain these goals; short-term goals need to be attainable/realistic (and no more than 3 goals) and expressed in a positive way:

Short-term goals (specific, measurable goals; no more than 3 goals)	Specific strategies, techniques, or actions to achieve the goal

2) MENTAL ROUTINES

Mental routines use a combination of mental conditioning tools (i.e. imagery, self-talk, relaxation) to help athletes enhance or prepare for performance. Types of routines include A) pre-competition; B) in-game (pre-performance, between-play, & post-performance); and C) post-competition.

A) Pre-competition (or pre-practice) Routine

Being prepared mentally for a competition involves focus, confidence, positive attitude, and feeling relaxed. An effective pre-competition routine often uses a combination of tools including breathing, positive self-talk, and imagery and is practiced regularly for reinforcement. Music can affect arousal regulation, concentration, mood enhancement, and team cohesion. Incorporating it into the pre-game routine may enhance individual and team performance.

Sample routine:

- Doing a cycle of deep-breathing can be calming if excessive arousal or anxiety is present. Deep-breathing can also facilitate focusing and staying in the present moment. Conversely, the fast-breathing exercise may be used to "psych-up" or get the energy level up (see pages 13 &

14 of the handbook for deep and fast breathing exercises).

- Music can be useful to either calm or energize an individual and to keep distractions outside one's mindset.

- Taking a moment to review strategy in your mind and visualize yourself executing plays successfully will help you get focused, confident, and ready for play.

- Feelings of confidence also may come through trusting the conditioning and other preparation that has been made during practice sessions of the preceding week.

- Staying loose and relaxed can be achieved through light, positive conversation with teammates while still maintaining a focus on the present situation.

B) In-Game Routines

In-game routines, or routines used during the course of play, include pre-performance, between-play, and post-performance.

Pre-performance Routine

The pre-performance routine precedes the beginning of a shot or play. It is used in sporting activities where there are breaks which allow the athlete a brief moment of preparation (e.g. between serves in tennis; prior to a free throw in basketball). These routines can be effective for focus and distraction and can be further enhanced if a tactile component is attached (e.g. prior to a free throw, holding and bouncing the basketball). Steps in the pre-performance routine include:

- Readying— coping skills are used to create a setting of self-confidence, focus, and emotional control.

- Imaging— successful execution is imaged.

- Focusing attention externally— attention is focused on a meaningful outside cue or thought.

- Calm execution— staying calm and thinking positively as the skill is executed.

If time allows, the execution and outcome of the skill as

well as pre-performance routine can also be assessed.

Between-play Routine

The between-play routine is used during breaks in play action such as between games in tennis or during a pitching change in softball. During this time, it is important to remain positive and relaxed but also still present in the moment. Breathing, self-talk, and imaging are tools useful during this period.

Example: Softball outfielders, who have seen no action in the game to this point, are waiting for a pitching change.

Mental routine: Given the players' inaction, doing things to remain psyched-up or energized may be indicated. A round of quick breathing can be effective to stay energized in addition to engaging in positive, energizing self-talk or chatter with teammates. Reminding oneself of strategy important for the moment and visualizing oneself in position and executing successful play can keep one focused and confident.

Post-performance Routine

The term, post-performance routine, is used here to describe the period immediately following the execution of a skill (as opposed to the time following a match or game which is referred to as post-competition). It can be helpful to have a routine if one has trouble under pressure or has difficulty shaking-off a negative outcome following executing a skill.

Example:

Researchers have found, for example that golfers who excelled under pressure, performed a consistent post-performance routine after each shot. The routine included a positive thought or reflection followed by a deliberate, physical action that served as a trigger for directing attention toward the next shot. In other words, following each shot, the successful golfers took a moment to find and think about the positive in the situation despite the negative outcome (e.g. "My ball did not hit the preferred spot, but it also did not hit the sand trap"). Following this reflection they would remove their glove (deliberate physical, behavioral response) that triggered their attention to be directed toward the next shot.

C) Post-Competition Routine

The post-competition period immediately follows the conclusion of the game or match. A mental routine during this time may include taking a moment to reflect on positives that can be taken away from the overall performance. A detailed, critical analysis should be saved for the next practice session. In addition, having something positive to do after the game, as a distraction to take your mind away from the field or court, is recommended (e.g. having dinner with family or friends not involved in sports; watching a funny movie, etc).

3) MENTAL CONDITIONING TIPS & EXERCISES

a) Staying focused.

Focus in the moment. Breathing (e.g. taking a quick breath or a slow, deep breath) can help you re-set and ready your mind for play in the moment or between moments (*for breathing exercises, see page 13 & 14 of the guide*).   In addition, reciting to yourself an active word or phrase such as "focus" or "attack" can reorient your attention to the task at hand.

The brain actually works best when you tell it what to do rather than what not to do. Therefore, during play, focus on what you DO want to happen instead of what you don't want to happen. For example, telling yourself, "I want the ball to land in left field" is more productive than saying, "I hope I don't hit the ball into foul territory."

Shifting from off to on the playing field. The "mental locker" exercise can help you switch from being preoccupied with issues off the field to being focused on the field.   When you arrive to the locker room, you start by opening an imaginary "mental locker." As you undress, the removal of each piece of clothing (e.g. coat, shirt, pants, shoe) represents the discarding of a problem or personal concern. For example, taking off your coat and putting it away in the locker may represent temporarily putting away the disagreement you had with your girlfriend that morning. In other words, the act of attaching a problem to an item of street clothing, physically shedding it, and replacing it with your uniform (which is associated with the game) can help you set aside a problem in the short term and focus on the game.

b) Displacing negative self-talk. We all have self-talk or conversations that run in our heads like an audiotape. The self-talk in an athlete's head can be competing voices, one that is positive and supportive and one that is negative and critical. The athlete has a CHOICE as to which voice he or she listens to. Remaining conscious of this choice is important. What kind of tape runs in your head? Is the negative voice stronger than the positive voice? Stay conscious of choosing the voice that provides and reinforces positive thoughts.

c) Turning negatives into positives. To turn negatives into positives you should view your setbacks or disappointments as temporary rather than permanent. Compartmentalize the problems (i.e. put them in a "box") and don't let them distract or affect every area of your life. In addition, internalize your victories (e.g. through constantly replaying in your mind your best moments) and externalize your defeats by thinking forward to the future (e.g. "That loss was just one game. It's over and time to move forward. I know what I need to work on to be better for the next game").

d) Diffusing pressure. Some athletes decrease pressure by thinking of something pleasant that they can look forward to after the game. For example, looking forward to being with family or having a few days off where you can go home and go fishing, hiking, hunting, etc.

Some athletes use indifference to their advantage. That is, they know that they have prepared and trained hard and can't be any more ready for the moment. At this point they trust their training and let "whatever happens, happen." The hard training is over, there is nothing to lose, so they allow themselves to let go and enjoy the moment.

When athletes are under pressure they often tense up and over-try (which can lead to a poor performance). It's important to find ways to physically relax. Some athletes use deep breathing and progressive muscle relaxation to calm themselves mentally. *For deep breathing and progressive muscle relaxation exercises, see page 13 & 15 of the guide.*

e) **Goal-setting**. When setting goals, make them very specific, measurable, and observable. Clearly identify a time frame for attaining the goals. Make the goals of moderate difficulty level (i.e. not too easy or hard). Write your goals down and monitor the progress (keep a journal). Use a mix of goals (i.e. a performance goal such as scoring 20 points in a basketball game and a process goal such as bending wrist and following through as you shoot the ball). Break down a long-term goal into a series of smaller goals (i.e. "baby steps"). Set practice as well as competition goals. Share your goals – this helps you stay committed and allows others to hold you accountable. *For a specific exercise that can help you outline new short-term and long-term goals see pages 31-33 of the guide.*

f) **Daily learning & growth**. It's important to invest in daily learning and to understand how what you've learned today will improve your performance tomorrow. Focus on the process of understanding yourself and improving your weaknesses rather than on outcomes.

g) Staying committed. There is no substitute for commitment to hard work. Once a commitment is made to putting the hours and effort in, success will follow. There's no getting around it - to succeed there needs to be a real commitment. Ask yourself, "how bad do I really want this?"

h) Avoiding self-defeating distractions. It's important to follow your goals and not what others do. Be strong enough to step back from trouble and self-defeating situations. It helps to associate with people who will make you better. Plan ahead. For example, plan before going out. Visualize what you will and won't do at a social gathering (e.g. "I'll have 2 drinks maximum"). Set a specific time when you leave and stick to it. ("I'm out by midnight..."). Arrange ahead of time how you will get to and from a party safely and without putting yourself at risk.

i) Managing fear. *Facing fears*. It's important to accept fear and view it as a signal that is meant to get you energized. Fear tends to be a false belief that appears real. What are you afraid of? Does the fear interfere with your athletic performance? With your life in general? What thoughts, feelings, and physical sensations accompany the fear? Don't let fear scare you. Make a fearful situation familiar and therefore less overwhelming by repeatedly putting yourself in the situation during practice. If, for example, you fear embarrassment and shame from missing free throws during a game, repeatedly practice being in the situation. Practice the situation in your mind repeatedly. This will make the actual situation feel less dreadful and threatening. See yourself walking up to the line confidently, not worried about the crowd or the outcome of the shot. Focus on executing the best technique you can. Visualize yourself and go through the physical motions of executing the proper technique. Positive outcomes follow good technique. Rehearse this repeatedly as you shoot real free throws in practice and use the same imagery during games.

Fear of failure - Fear of failure or making mistakes can restrict a player and limit success. You should view failure as feedback. Be honest about your shortcomings, learn from them, and put the effort and energy into correcting them. Training harder and developing confidence and trust in your abilities can diffuse fear.

Fear of success - It's important to have a positive image of yourself. That is, seeing yourself succeeding and thinking of yourself as one who deserves to succeed. Visualize a moment of success in the past - this can reinforce that you're capable of succeeding. Be willing to take a risk in order to succeed; visualize yourself winning as a result of taking a risk.

j) Staying motivated. Motivation only comes from within. Most people are motivated to pursue the things they view as pleasurable. What is pleasurable to you about your sport at this point in time? About your training at this point in time? Does a fire burn within you? Do you have a mission? What is your mission at this point in time? What is your passion at this point? Write yourself a reminder of what motivates you and keep it in a place where you can see it regularly.

k) Riding the bench. If you are currently riding the bench, a way to stay actively engaged is to make a list of things you CAN do as opposed to can't do. Your list may include things such as studying film, staying on track with workouts, and supporting and cheering on teammates who are in the game. During game-time stay attentive to each play, as though you will be going into the game. Have a sense about and visualize what you might do in each play. Stay in the game mentally.

l) Taking responsibility. Know and be honest about who you are and the role your attitude plays in your success. Am I reliable? Does my attitude help my game or get in the way? Do I take responsibility for my choices and actions or do I blame others for my difficulties?

m) Controlling emotions. The most successful athletes are those who control their emotions. Be aware that you can't always control what happens (e.g. in a game or in life in general) but you can control how you respond to a situation. In instances where you feel frustrated, ask yourself, what factors can I control in this situation? What factors can't I control? How can I respond in a way that is not self-defeating? Before you can control your performance, you must be in control of yourself.

n) Building self-belief & confidence. Research supports that our subconscious mind plays a major role in how we view and actualize our lives and that it can be influenced by what we actively think and say to ourselves. Positive, affirming self-talk (i.e. self-affirming statements or "affirmations") can be used to "re-program" the subconscious mind to encourage us to believe in ourselves.

Affirmations are statements that are meant to create self-belief and self-change. They can serve as inspiration, simple reminders, or as triggers to focus attention on goals throughout the day that promote positive, sustained self-belief and change. Effective affirmations are stated in first person. Always start your affirmation with "I" or "I am..." This turns an affirmation into a statement of identity which is a powerful motivator for self-belief and change.

Always state your affirmations in the positive. For example, instead of saying, "I no longer enjoy junk food," you might say, "I am free from junk food," or "I am a healthy person and I love the way my body feels when I make healthy choices."

Write your affirmations in the present state, as if they are already happening. For example, affirm to yourself, "I am fit and strong," instead of "Eight weeks from now, I will be fit and strong."

Attach strong feeling and emotion to your affirmations, as there is a strong link between emotion words and behavior. So, instead of "I only eat healthy food," which sounds chore-like, say "I feel vibrant and alive when I make healthy choices for me."

In addition, self-affirming statements should be realistic, achievable, and REHEARSED REGULARLY.

Confidence comes not only from self-belief but also from preparation which includes a mental plan. The best athletes visualize not only best-case but also worst case scenarios. They don't imagine failing but plan how they may handle a difficult situation. When preparing, leave nothing undone. No detail is too small. Visualization is helpful in this situation. For example, a softball pitcher may visualize how she is going to pitch to each hitter, seeing and feeling the physical sensation of throwing exactly the pitches she wants to throw. She may go through the entire line-up in detail a few times in her mind. Before even stepping on the field, her opponents feel familiar and less threatening and her confidence is heightened.

o) **Having trust & consistency**. Successful athletes trust their talent. Trust comes from having awareness of your natural talents and training hard to develop them. Consistent preparation leads to consistent performance. Think, act, and practice with consistency and then trust your talent and preparation.

p) **Role of superstitions**. Superstitions are based more on the idea of luck than on a mental strategy. When an athlete has a superstition, he or she is relying on certain objects such as a pair of socks or a hair ribbon to bring positive results in their performance. Superstitions are not a reliable strategy because the athlete is not in direct control of the outcome, however they do put the athlete in a positive mind set to perform. Superstitions when used as more of a routine, for example eating a favorite cereal every morning, can help the athlete stay focused and relaxed.

q) Pre-game warm-up. It is known that athletes (of equal abilities) who utilize mental conditioning outperform those who don't. Many athletes use imagery (e.g. visualization) to mentally warm-up prior to competitive play.

Some individuals even go to the extent of creating a "mind-space" or imaginary place where they "enter" and perform their mental warmup. For example, prior to a game, the athlete may find a quiet corner, lay or sit in a comfortable position, close his eyes, and enter his mental retreat where he will do his mental warm-up. First, he recalls details of one of his best performances, re-experiencing the winning feeling from that moment. He relives not only the visual images but also, sounds, smells, and physical sensations associated with the moment. Then he lets those images go and starts rehearsing for the upcoming game. For example, he sees himself, during the game, executing successful moves past defenders and with teammates on offense. A quarterback may review in his mind defenses he saw on film and is likely to see from his opponent during the game. A baseball player may review pitches he is likely to see from the opposing starting pitcher.

Having prepared, not only physically but also mentally, allows you to leave the field after the game knowing you did all you could do to be ready to compete that

day. This satisfaction creates a sense of pride which can
be motivation to prepare on a consistent basis.

III. GENERAL MENTAL HEALTH

MENTAL WELLNESS, BALANCE, & LIFE SKILLS

Mental Wellness & Balance

Mental wellness has been defined as a state of emotional and psychological well-being in which an individual is able to use his or her cognitive and emotional capabilities, function in society, and meet the ordinary demands of everyday life. There are many theories regarding what constitutes a "balanced" life but many suggest that connecting with others, making time for yourself, having hobbies you enjoy, practicing healthy habits, practicing gratitude, and helping others are means to being a balanced individual. Creating balance in life contributes significantly to mental wellness.

Elite athletes value balance and agree that success involves not only intense focus, hard work, and commitment to their sport, but also engagement and investment in activities and relationships outside of sport. In addition, the concept of "having fun" while preparing for or in the midst of competition plays a key role in success.

Life Skills & Student-Athletes

Developing an armamentarium of "life skills" is a way to create and maintain a healthy, balanced life. Life skills has been described as a foundation of abilities which include self-awareness, problem-solving, decision-making, time-management, communication, and the ability to cope with stress. The skills needed to succeed in sports are essentially the same as those needed to succeed in life.

During a student-athlete's college career, life skills are invaluable. They help individuals deal successfully with the daily demands of their studies as well as their sport disciplines. In addition, the sports setting offers athletes another place to practice and perfect life skills.

Transition to a life beyond college and sports can be difficult. In order to manage it smoothly, individuals must believe that they have skills and qualities that are of value in other settings. In addition, they must have assistance in developing these abilities.

A life skills curriculum, integrated into an academic institution's athletics program, assists student-athletes in developing skills that can be utilized both during and beyond their college careers. Student-athletes utilizing support are more likely to find interest and value in school (which can affect motivation to graduate). They potentially leave with greater knowledge, skills, confidence, emotional grounding, and experience. Academic institutions benefit as well, having the opportunity to mentor students, develop productive citizens, and achieve educational missions and graduation success.

Specific topics commonly addressed in collegiate life skills programs

1) Finance management.

2) Time management.

3) Stress management.

4) Resume writing.

5) Interview skills.

6) Conflict management.

7) Dressing for success.

8) Etiquette.

9) Goal setting.

10) Healthy relationships.

11) Mental health awareness.

12) Drug/alcohol abuse awareness.

13) Maintaining healthy habits (e.g. nutrition, hygiene).

III. GENERAL MENTAL HEALTH

PSYCHOSOCIAL ISSUES IN THE SPORTS SETTING

1) Team Cohesion

The concept of group cohesion, defined as a dynamic process in which a group strives to form and remain together in the pursuit of goals and objectives, applies similarly to the concept of team cohesion. Teams may go through stages in order to become a cohesive unit:

1. Forming stage– there is enthusiasm about new relationships and getting together for a common purpose.
2. Storming stage– there is struggle and frustration in trying to learn a new system and interact with others who are dissimilar.
3. Norming stage– there is agreement about what the common goals and parameters of what acceptable and good performance entails.
4. Performing stage– the team interacts in-sync and performs as a cohesive unit.

For a team to work optimally as a unit, there must be self-motivation and a sense of personal satisfaction among individuals and good communication among team members. Benefits of team cohesion include not only improved performance, but also improved mood and emotions for individuals, team confidence and momentum, and motivation among individuals to participate in subsequent sporting activity.

Interventions to Promote Team Cohesion (for Coaches or Team Leaders)

Team cohesion may be promoted in the following ways:

1. Acquainting each player with the responsibility of other teammates (e.g. playing one another's positions).
2. Having some personal knowledge about each player (e.g. have a sense about one's interests outside of sports).
3. Developing pride among team subunits (e.g. defensive squad pride vs offensive squad pride in football).
4. Allowing individuals to feel like the team is theirs and not the coach's.
5. Setting clear goals and achieving them.
6. Helping individual members learn and value his or her role.
7. Not expecting total social harmony.
8. Having team drills prior to a game that encourage group cooperation.
9. Highlighting moments of success.
10. Believing that the team can and will succeed.
11. Not creating too much competition among team members.
12. Educating the team about destructive factors such as clique formation & jealousy.

2) Managing Team Conflict

On occasion, conflicts among team members will occur. Conflict often begins through a difference in people's behaviors, interests, desires, or values. It can also begin through jealousy or personal dislike of other's values.

Negative effects of conflict on a team may include: team members feeling defeated, demoralized, anxious, stressed, or inadequate; development of a distrustful or suspicious environment; disrupted communication resulting in a lack of cooperation and information not being conveyed; poor work and team relationships; and a decline in performance.

On the other hand, resolution of conflicts has the following positive effects on a team: increased motivation and creativity (i.e. new ideas as new approaches are sought); clarification of issues and ideas; improved team performance and cohesion; improved tolerance among players; increased trust; and increased sense of achievement.

Resolving conflict begins with recognizing both positive and negative team behavior and then taking actions to outline a solution to the problem. When dealing with conflict with other teammates, it is important to first and foremost not make the situation worse. Behaviors associated with inflaming conflict include:

1. Blaming others.

2. Only valuing your opinion and no one else's.

3. Insulting others.

4. Waging verbal threats and ultimatums.

5. Getting defensive.

6. Avoiding or running away from the problem.

7. Beating around the bush or talking around the point.

8. Telling others instead of the source; talking behind one's back.

9. Inflammatory social media messages.

10. Making assumptions about others instead of understanding the true circumstances.

Constructive ways to manage conflict include:

1. Staying in control of your own emotions.

2. Stating your concerns clearly, supporting what you say with facts, and expressing yourself in a respectful tone and manner.

3. Addressing the conflict with the other party directly.

4. Working with other team members to outline a solution to the problem.

5. Actively listening or demonstrating that you care about resolving the problem and that you care about what others have to say.

6. Remaining positive and assuming that the other has good intentions for resolving the issue as well.

3) Coping with Injury

Injuries are often an unavoidable aspect of participating in athletics. Psychological and emotional reactions to athletic injuries will vary from one individual to the next. Factors influencing one's response include type of injury, severity of injury, and the coping mechanisms used by the athlete. Athletes who experience high levels of stress (on or off the field) tend to be at greater risk of being injured.

It is important for athletes, trainers, team physicians, and coaching staff to understand normal and maladaptive emotional reactions to injury. Normal reactions may include frustration, sadness, anger, irritability, decreased motivation, disengagement, and even changes in sleep and appetite. If these feelings grow more intense or persistent, particularly to the point of impairing one's function, a more significant mental condition may be present (e.g. adjustment disorders, major depression). In addition, an increased risk for maladaptive behavior such as disordered eating and substance abuse may occur. In extreme cases, suicidal or self-injurious thoughts may occur.

Individuals with limited coping skills or poor adjustment may struggle with reluctance to seek support. Some with coping limitations avoid revealing their emotions for fear of appearing weak while those with a problematic sense of entitlement may have difficulty accepting and dealing appropriately with adversity or failure.   In addition, many young athletes have not developed their identities outside of being an athlete. If their identity as an athlete is threatened by injury or illness, they may experience a significant feeling of "loss."

Warning signs indicating poor adjustment to injuries include unreasonable fear of re-injury, ongoing denial of injury, severity and response to recovery, general impatience and irritability, rapid mood swings, social withdrawal, extreme guilt about disappointing the team, focusing on minor physical complaints, and preoccupation with the question of return-to-play.

Interventions

Most emotional responses by athletes to an injury are transient. The athletic healthcare team (trainers, team doctors) and social support network (family, friends, teammates) are often effective in helping the athlete deal with emotional issues. Nevertheless, athletes with problematic psychological reactions who need treatment should seek care through a licensed mental health professional (ideally one experienced in working with athletes).

Psychological strategies such as goal setting, positive self-statements, cognitive restructuring, and imagery/visualization have been associated with faster recovery. Healthy coping for injuries has included accepting responsibility for the injury; being knowledgeable about the injury and taking an active part in self-care; keeping a positive attitude; using a support network of friends and family; setting appropriate and achievable goals; maintaining levels of fitness while injured (as approved by the coaching and healthcare staffs); and being patient.

4) Career Termination

Career termination (i.e. ending one's career in competitive athletics) is a significant event in an athlete's life. Reasons for ending a career in sports may include advanced age (resulting in an inability to physically perform effectively), deselection (being cut or not being chosen to participate as an active member of the team), injury, and free choice.

Factors affecting an athlete's ability to adapt to career termination include:

A) General social and psychological development— e.g. development of well-rounded interests and healthy coping mechanisms in youth;

B) Self-identity—defining one's identity and self-worth solely in terms of his or her athletic activities and achievements is associated with suffering identity issues and negative consequences;

C) Social identity—when athletes retire, there may be a loss of social identity and social status;

D) Sense of control—those who perceive that they are in control of the decision to exit are less likely to experience a difficult transition compared to those who perceive they are not in control;

E) Other factors - e.g. socioeconomic status and

capacity to access stable financial resources will also impact a successful transition out of sports.

Coping strategies, social support, and pre-retirement planning are resources often used by athletes adapting to career transition. Examples of coping strategies include thinking and talking about eventual retirement **early** in one's career; maintaining contact with friends and acquaintances in the athletic community; and maintaining a regular workout schedule. Having a strong social support network outside of athletics can provide individuals with a constructive, well-rounded perspective and make the transition from sport into non-sport life smoother. Regarding pre-retirement planning, those athletes who are able to meet with a consultant before they retire are more likely to find alternative career opportunities than those who do not.

Poor adaptation to career termination has been associated with substance abuse, criminal activity, and mental health issues (e.g. depression, anxiety, adjustment disorders). Psychiatric conditions should be evaluated and treated by a certified mental health professional.

III. GENERAL MENTAL HEALTH

OTHER MENTAL CONDITIONS ASSOCIATED WITH SPORTS

1) Normal Anxiety & Anxiety Disorders

Anxiety may be defined as a state of neurological arousal characterized by both physical and psychological signs. Anxiety may be a normal reaction that acts as a signal to the body that aspects of its systems are under stress.

Common signs of anxiety are outlined in the table below:

Physical signs	Psychological signs
Headache	Feeling of dread
Muscle tension	Poor concentration
Back pain	Impaired sleep
Abdominal pain	Impaired sexual desire
Tremulousness or "shakiness"	
Fatigue	
Numbness	
Shortness of breath	
Palpitations	
Sweating	
Hyper-vigilant reflexes (i.e. easily startled; "jumpy")	

Anxiety "disorders" are considered when the signals triggered by the body produce prolonged physical or psychological discomfort or a pattern and degree of distress that disrupts normal function.   Collectively, anxiety disorders are the most common mental disorder in the United States (US), affecting 18% of the adult population age 18 and older. Anxiety disorders are one of the most common mental health problems on college campuses with nearly half of US college students having experienced overwhelming anxiety in the last year.

Performance anxiety (social anxiety disorder), panic disorder, and phobic anxiety following injury are more common types of anxiety disorders found in athletes. Generalized anxiety and obsessive-compulsive disorder (OCD) are less common. Each of these conditions is described in this section.

Anxiety Disorders in Athletes

A) Social Anxiety Disorder (social phobia; performance anxiety)

A persistent, unreasonable fear of one or more social or performance situations in which the person is exposed to unfamiliar people or to possible scrutiny by others. The individual fears that he or she will act in a way (or show anxiety symptoms) that will be embarrassing and humiliating. The feared situations are avoided or else are endured with intense anxiety and distress.

B) Panic Disorder

Panic disorder involves a sudden, spontaneous onset of overwhelming anxiety symptoms.

C) Phobia

An irrational fear of a particular object or situation causing anxiety symptoms.

D) Generalized Anxiety Disorder (GAD)

GAD is defined as anxiety that persists constantly throughout the day and occurs chronically over time.

E) Obsessive-Compulsive Disorder (OCD)

The presence of obsessions (i.e. constant intrusive thoughts or urges causing anxiety symptoms) and/or compulsions (i.e. unusual and excessive behaviors or mental acts one is compelled to perform repetitively in order to reduce anxiety to a dreaded situation or event).

Management of anxiety disorders

Outlined below are a few exercises that may be useful in decreasing some forms of anxiety. More extensive psychotherapeutic interventions provided by a certified mental health professional may be indicated depending on the type of anxiety disorder and the severity of symptoms (e.g. cognitive-behavioral therapy, medication therapy).

A) *Breathing and progressive relaxation* have been effective for reducing anxiety (e.g. performance anxiety or social anxiety, panic disorder, phobia, generalized anxiety). These techniques are outlined in detail on pages 12-16 of this book.

B) *Graded exposure (i.e. gradual re-exposure to a feared situation or object feared)* may be particularly useful for phobias. It incorporates the breathing and relaxation exercises as well. The key strategy for overcoming fears of this kind involves creating a graded plan or hierarchy of steps. The individual is gradually exposed to the fearful object or situation, in small steps, so that eventually less anxiety is experienced when the object or situation is present. Tools such as breathing, positive self-talk, and imagery (i.e. visualization) may be used to reduce the anxiety felt during moments when an aspect of the frightening object or situation is present.

Example: A diver has anxiety and a fear of diving after an incident where she hit her head on the platform and sustained a concussion. Using graded exposure, the diver first gradually gets herself to climb the ladder to the platform; then to stand on the platform edge; then to jump into the water; and then to perform progressively more difficult dives into the water. At each step in the process, she uses 1) breathing to calm herself physically and 2) positive self-talk and imagery (of successful execution in the past) for confidence and motivation.

C) *Problem-solving exercise*

(May be especially useful for performance anxiety & generalized anxiety).

Choose one or two problems that are particularly bothersome and make a decision to try to resolve them as best as possible.

1. On a sheet of paper, list the specific problems.

2. List five or six possible solutions to each problem. Write down any ideas that occur to you, not merely the "good" ideas.

3. Evaluate the positive and negative points of each idea.

4. Choose the solution that best fits your needs.

5. Plan exactly the steps you will take to put the solution into action.

6. Review your efforts after attempting to carry out the plan. Praise all efforts. If unsuccessful, start again.

D) *Managing negative, distorted thinking*

(May be especially useful for performance anxiety, generalized anxiety, and obsessive -compulsive disorder).

Significant anxiety can influence thoughts and emotions and progress to negative, pessimistic feelings and even irrational, distorted thoughts.

Management of negative, distorted thoughts involves:

- Identifying the negative, distorted thoughts.

- Substituting these thoughts with more realistic ideas (create a list of alternative thoughts that are realistic, positive and counter each negative thought listed). This is an important skill that can help reduce anxiety symptoms.

2) Major Depression

Major depression has been generally described as a decline in mood that persists for an extended period, represents a decrease from a previous level of function, and causes some impairment in function. It is one of the most common mental disorders in the United States (US). An estimated 6.7% of all adults in the US aged 18 or older had at least one major depressive episode in the past year. Approximately one-third of college students have experienced impaired function in the last 12 months due to depression. In addition, more than 30% of students who have a history of utilizing mental health services have seriously considered attempting suicide at some point in their lives.

Circumstances related to sports in which athletes may develop depression include injury, poor athletic performance, over-training (where one can become not only physically, but also emotionally exhausted), and transition out of a life of regular sports activity (such as upon graduation from college or the end of a professional career). In addition, having depression may lead to poor athletic performance and increase one's risk for getting injured.

Signs & Characteristics of Depression

- Persistent depressed mood and loss of pleasure in activities that normally give pleasure.

- Weight loss or gain.

- Insomnia (i.e. too little sleep) or hypersomnia (i.e. too much sleep).

- Psychomotor agitation (i.e. agitated movement) or retardation (i.e. slowed movement).

- Energy loss.

- Feelings of worthlessness or guilt.

- Poor concentration or memory; indecisiveness.

- Hopelessness or suicidal thoughts with the intention to act or with specific plans made.

Management of Depression

There is no shame in feeling depressed. It can be helpful to identify those individuals who can serve as strong supports and to use them during periods of distress (e.g. family, friends, coaches, clergy, mental health professionals). When dealing with challenging situations, staying positive, staying in touch with your strengths, and focusing on what you can control can be helpful. Psychotherapy and, in severe cases, medication therapy provided by certified mental health professionals are significantly effective for the treatment of depression. A mental health professional should be consulted immediately if there are ever feelings of severe hopelessness or suicidality.

3) Substance Use Disorders

A psychoactive substance may be defined as any substance that can activate the brain and cause effects on thoughts, emotions, and behaviors. A substance use disorder may be characterized as a condition that involves the continuous use of a psychoactive substance or substances in a pathological pattern that adversely affects mental health, physical health, and social function. According to the U.S. Surgeon General, over 20 million people in the United States have a substance use disorder.

Definitions

1. Intoxication – maladaptive behavior associated with recent drug ingestion.

2. Withdrawal – adverse physical & psychological symptoms that occur following cessation of the drug.

3. Tolerance – the need for more substance to attain the same level of effect.

4. Pathological use (also referred to as abuse) – a maladaptive pattern of use leading to repetitive problems and negative consequences (i.e. use in dangerous situations such as driving; use leading to

legal, social, and occupational problems).

5. Misuse— the use a drug for a purpose for which it is not intended (e.g. taking a prescribed narcotic pain medication, such as oxycontin, for anxiety or insomnia).

6. Dependence (addiction) — continued desire for and use of a psychoactive substance to satisfy pleasurable urges and/or to alleviate the effects of withdrawal. Dependence may be psychological or physical in nature.

Psychological dependence:

- Persistent substance use, despite evidence of its harmful consequences.

- Difficulties in controlling the use of the substance.

- Neglect of interests and an increased amount of time taken to obtain the substance or recover from its effects.

- Evidence of tolerance such that higher doses are required to achieve the same effect.

- Compulsion or craving - a strong desire to take the substance.

- Anxiety or mood disturbance occurs if the drug is not taken.

Physical dependence:

- Physical symptoms occur if the drug is not taken (e.g. headache; gastrointestinal distress; changes in blood pressure, heart rate; sweating; tremors; muscular pain).

Alcohol

According to the Surgeon General, alcohol misuse contributes to approximately 88,000 deaths in the United States each year. Over 66 million people reported binge drinking in the past month. Alcohol use is fairly widespread among college students with approximately 4 of 5 students drinking and about half engaging in binge drinking (i.e. consumption of an excessive amount of alcohol in a short period of time). Negative consequences of alcohol abuse and misuse have included personal, work, or academic problems; health problems; unintentional injuries (and death from unintentional injuries); suicide attempts; being a victim of rape or other sexual abuse; and being a victim of assault.

Effects of Alcohol

Intoxication Symptoms: Slurred speech; unstable walking; mood change; aggression; anxiety; psychosis; sleep disturbance; and delirium.

Withdrawal Symptoms (occurring several hours to a few days after cessation of use that has been heavy and prolonged): Nausea; headache; nystagmus (rapid horizontal movement of eyeballs); unstable blood pressure or heart rate; psychosis; anxiety; mood disturbance; sleep disturbance; delirium; and seizure.

Effects on Athletic Performance

The effect of alcohol on athletic performance depends on the amount and type of alcohol ingested, the weight and health of the individual, and the timing of the alcohol consumption. Alcohol is a central nervous system (CNS) depressant and may cause decreased concentration, coordination, reaction time, strength, power, and endurance. Alcohol also can inhibit the body's absorption of nutrients vital for optimal performance.

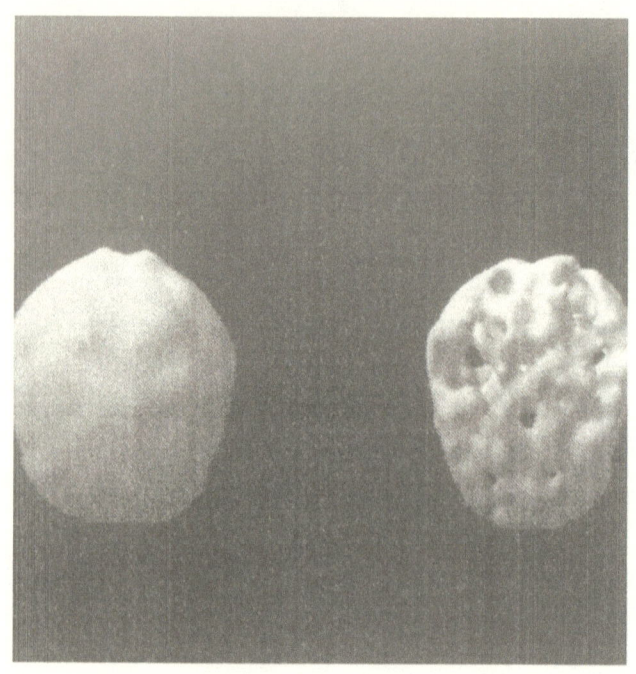

SPECT Scan of a Brain Affected by Alcohol.

SPECT stands for single photon emission computed tomography. While computerized tomography (CT or CAT) scans and magnetic resonance imaging (MRI) scans show what the brain actually physically looks like, SPECT looks at how the brain functions. That is, a SPECT scan can show how areas of the brain are more active or less active (i.e. providing data on brain blood flow and brain cell metabolism). Above, is a SPECT image which illustrates a normal brain (left image) vs a brain affected by alcohol use twice weekly on a regular basis (right image). "Holes" noted in the image of the alcohol brain are damaged regions with low blood flow and poor activity.

Cannabis (marijuana)

Marijuana is the most commonly used illicit drug with approximately 22.2 million users in the past month. Marijuana use has been on the rise and college students now smoke marijuana daily more often than they drink alcohol daily. Daily marijuana use among college students has more than tripled in the past two decades.

Effects of Cannabis

Tetrahydrocannabinol (THC) is the principal psychoactive component of cannabis. Intoxication symptoms of cannabis include elevated or depressed mood; anxiety; inappropriate laughing; paranoia; hallucinations; red eyes; increased appetite; dry mouth; and increased heart rate.

Withdrawal Symptoms (occurring 1 week after cessation of prolonged, heavy use, i.e. a few months of daily or near daily use) include depressed or irritable mood; anxiety; restlessness; sleep disturbance; poor appetite; and weight loss.

Studies have indicated an association between high doses of cannabis and delirium, panic, and ongoing psychosis. In addition, long-term use has been linked to anxiety, depression, and a loss of motivation.

Effects on Athletic Performance

The effects of marijuana on sport performance are similar to those of alcohol. Reduced reaction time, impaired motor and eye-hand coordination, and impaired time perception have been associated with cannabis use.

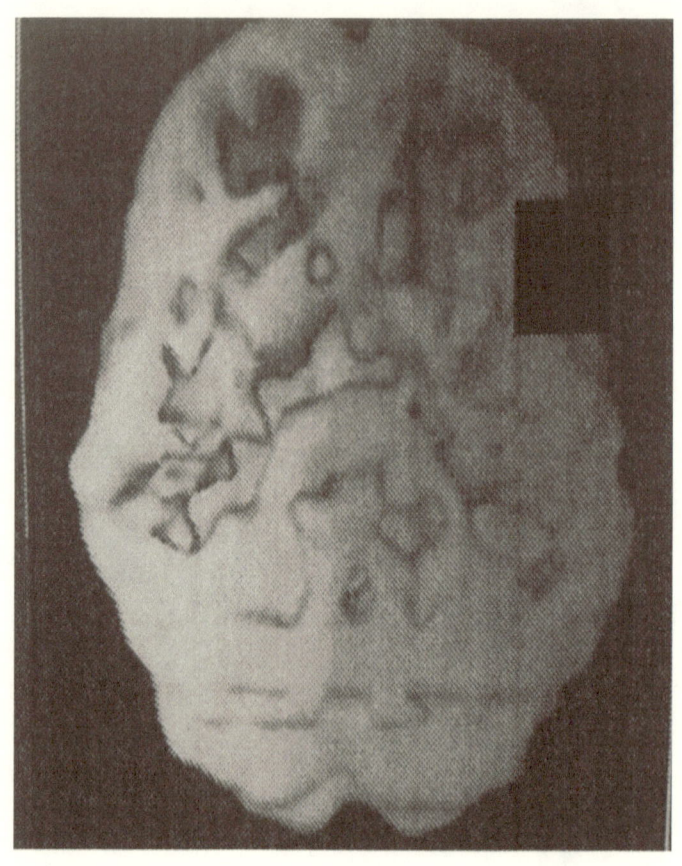

A SPECT image of a brain affected by cannabis use. "Holes" in the image indicate regions with low brain blood flow and cell activity.

Stimulants

Stimulants (drugs stimulating or activating the central nervous system) are a class of substance that includes amphetamines, methamphetamine, cocaine, ephedrine, and Attention Deficit-Hyperactivity Disorder (ADHD) medications such as Adderall or Ritalin. More than 12 million people in the United States (4.7 percent of the population) have tried methamphetamine at least once. Adults aged 18 to 25 years have a higher rate of current cocaine use than any other age group, with 1.4 percent of young adults reporting cocaine use in the past month. In the past year, an estimated 9.6% of full-time college students in the USA have used Adderall and 4.4% have used cocaine.

Effects of Stimulants

The most common effects of stimulants are euphoria and pleasure. Additional short term effects of stimulants include increased heart rate, increased body temperature, increased blood pressure, nausea, blurred vision, dilated pupils, confusion, and muscle spasms. Potential long term effects of stimulants may include anorexia or extreme weight loss, hallucinations, paranoia or anxiety, difficulty concentrating or focusing, and dental problems. Withdrawal may also occur with stimulants with symptoms including craving, depression, anxiety, extreme fatigue, sleep disturbance, vivid dreams, dehydration, dulled senses, jitteriness, hunger, impaired memory, and paranoia.

Effect on Athletic Performance

There are a number of adverse effects that stimulants may have on athletic performance. Skills requiring fine motor coordination can be negatively affected by tremulousness or jitteriness associated with stimulants. These drugs can also cause one to feel overly energetic, which may lead to overexertion and injury. Stimulants also may increase the risk for cardiovascular complications which can result in death.

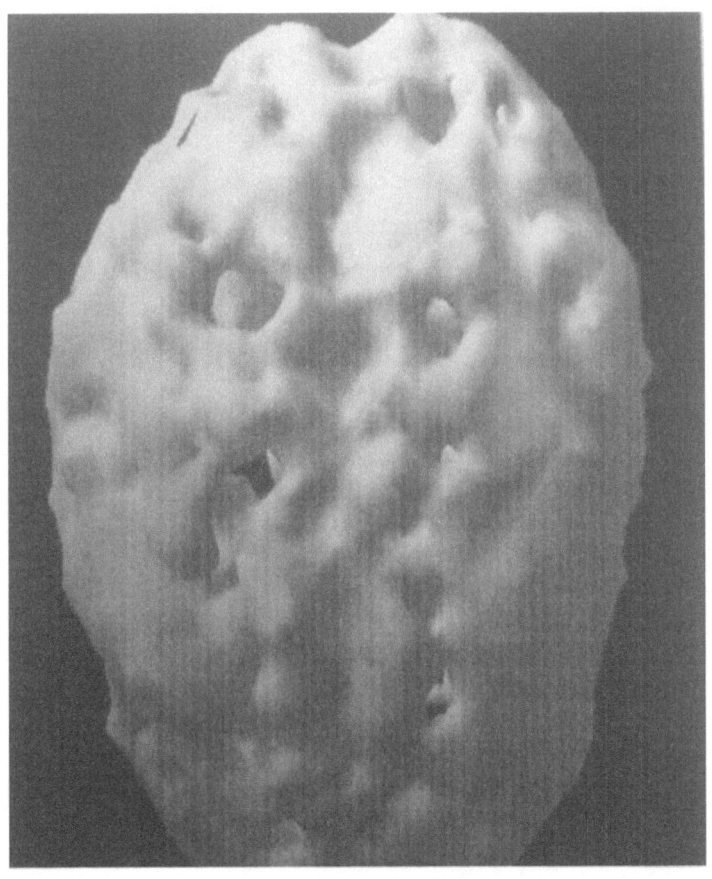

SPECT Scan of brain affected by stimulant (cocaine).
Again, "holes" in the image depict areas where brain
blood flow and activity are decreased.

Management of Substance Use Disorders

Evaluation by a medical or mental health professional will assure the proper assessment and management of symptoms and conditions related to substance use disorders. Detoxification, inpatient/outpatient rehabilitation, Alcoholics Anonymous (AA), and Narcotics Anonymous (NA) are some forms of treatment that are employed depending on the type and extent of substance use.

4) Eating Disorders

Eating disorders are characterized by serious disturbances in eating behavior and weight regulation. The most common disorders are anorexia nervosa, bulimia nervosa, and binge-eating. Eating disorders often coexist with other mental conditions including depression, substance abuse, and anxiety disorders. In the general US population, they tend to appear in the teens or young adulthood and occur in women and girls approximately 2.5 times greater than among men and boys. Eating disorders are common in college students with a greater prevalence in women.

Elements of the sport environment may increase one's risk for developing an eating disorder. Eating disorders are often triggered by dieting and exist more commonly in sports that emphasize diet, appearance, size, and weight requirements (e.g. wrestling, gymnastics, diving, lightweight rowing, and cross-country running). While eating disorders tend to be prevalent in female athletes, male athletes are also at risk.

Athletic performance may be significantly affected by the physical effects of eating disorders. Intense dieting can adversely affect maximal oxygen consumption and running speed for some athletes. Restricting caloric intake, particularly carbohydrates, limits an important energy source. The risk of muscle injury and weakness increases with inadequate protein intake and metabolism. Dysfunctional behavior associated with eating disorders such as induced vomiting and excessive exercise can lead to dehydration.

The Female Athlete Triad, i.e. disordered eating, amenorrhea (loss of menstruation), and loss of bone mass (osteopenia/osteoporosis), usually begins with disordered eating. Inadequate nutrition can cause insufficient energy to fuel the athlete's exercise and training and to maintain normal bodily processes related to general health, growth and development. When this occurs, the reproductive system shuts down to conserve energy. As a result, the body stops producing estrogen. Without estrogen, the body cannot build bone mass, leading to a loss of bone mineral density.

Anorexia nervosa

Anorexia is an eating disorder characterized by a low weight, fear of gaining weight, distorted perception of body weight, and inappropriate eating and weight control behavior.

Symptoms of anorexia nervosa include:

- Abnormally low body weight.
- Significant food restriction.
- Constant pursuit of thinness and unwillingness to maintain a normal or healthy weight.
- Intense fear of gaining weight.
- Distorted body image and self-esteem that is heavily influenced by perceptions of body weight and shape; a denial of the seriousness of low body weight.
- Lack of menstruation among girls and women.

Other physical symptoms and medical complications associated with chronic anorexia:

- Bone thinning (osteopenia or osteoporosis).
- Dry, yellowish skin and brittle hair and nails.
- Growth of fine hair all over the body (lanugo).
- Weakness, muscle wasting, and anemia.
- Severe constipation.

- Low blood pressure or slowed breathing and pulse; damage to the structure and function of the heart.
- Brain damage; multi-organ failure.
- Drop in internal body temperature, causing a person to feel cold all the time.
- Fatigue or sluggishness.
- Infertility.

Bulimia nervosa

Bulimia is an eating disorder characterized by 1) a lack of control over eating and 2) episodes of excessive eating (binge-eating) followed by inappropriate methods of weight control (i.e. self-induced vomiting or purging, abuse of laxatives and diuretics, and excessive exercise).

One with bulimia may appear normal weight or slightly overweight. However, individuals often fear gaining weight, desperately desire to lose weight, and are intensely dissatisfied with their body size and shape. Bulimic behavior is typically done in secret and is often accompanied by feelings of disgust or shame. The binge eating and purging cycle can happen anywhere from several times a week to many times a day.

Physical symptoms associated with bulimia include:

- Sore, inflamed throat.
- Swollen salivary glands in the neck and jaw area.
- Tooth decay due to stomach acid from vomiting; worn tooth enamel.
- Acid reflux disorder and other gastrointestinal problems.
- Irritated bowels due to laxative abuse.
- Severe dehydration from purging of fluids.

- Electrolyte imbalance—too low or too high levels of sodium, calcium, potassium, and other minerals that can lead to a heart attack or seizures.

Binge-eating disorder

Binge-eating disorder is defined as recurrent binge or excessive eating episodes where one feels a loss of control over his or her eating. Feelings of guilt, shame, and distress about the binge-eating, (which can lead to more binge-eating) can occur. Unlike bulimia, binge-eating episodes are not followed by compensatory behaviors such as purging, excessive exercise, or fasting. Consequently, people with binge-eating disorder often are overweight or obese.

Management of Eating Disorders

Management of eating disorders involves restoring adequate nutrition, bringing weight to a healthy level, decreasing excessive exercise, and stopping binging and purging behaviors. Specific types of psychotherapy, or talk therapy have proven to be effective for eating disorders. Antidepressant medications may be effective for bulimia nervosa and co-occurring anxiety or depression for other eating disorders.

Treatment is tailored to the individual and may include:

- Individual, group, or family psychotherapy.
- Medical care and monitoring.
- Nutritional counseling.
- Medications (for example, antidepressants).
- Hospitalization for some patients who are severely malnourished or underweight.

5) Concussion

In simple terms, a concussion may be described as a disturbance in brain function caused by direct or indirect force to the head. A significant risk factor for concussion is having a prior concussion. If athletes already received one concussion, they are 1-2 times more likely to receive a second one. If they've had two concussions, a third is 2-4 times more likely, and if they've had three concussions, they are 3-9 times more likely to receive a fourth concussion. One with a history of developmental disorders, psychiatric disorders, or a history of headaches or migraines may be at risk for impaired recovery time after sustaining a concussion. Sustaining a concussion, having more symptoms, and requiring a greater recovery time have been associated with female athletes. However, it has also been indicated that, of NCAA athletes sustaining a sports-related concussion, the average number of symptoms and symptom resolution time does not differ by sex.

Symptoms

Symptoms of a concussion may be physical (e.g. headaches, dizziness, nausea), cognitive (e.g. difficulty with attention, concentration, or memory), or emotional (e.g. irritability, sadness). Disturbances in sleep, appetite, and energy levels may also occur. It has been indicated that a larger proportion of concussions in male college athletes tend to include amnesia and disorientation, while a larger proportion of concussions in female college athletes tend to include headache, nausea & vomiting, and excessive drowsiness.

Conditions Associated with Multiple Concussions

Multiple concussions have been associated with adverse conditions including:

1) Mild Cognitive Impairment (MCI) – involves impaired memory (and possibly other cognitive functions such as problem solving, decision making, word-finding) but is not severe enough to significantly impair daily function. MCI can be a sign of progression to dementia (when due to Alzheimer's Disease, for example). However, other causes of MCI may not cause progression to dementia and some may even be amenable to treatment.

2) Post-Concussion Syndrome – characterized by persistent symptoms (lasting 3 months or longer). Symptoms may include headache, dizziness, sleep disturbances, anxiety, cognitive problems (e.g. memory, concentration, etc), and changes in mood (depression or irritability).

3) Chronic Traumatic Encephalopathy (CTE) – a progressive neurodegenerative disease related to trauma to the brain. It is usually diagnosed after death and is a disease distinct from other conditions such as Alzheimer's Disease. Signs and symptoms associated with CTE include impaired cognition (memory, attention, judgment and evaluation, reasoning, computation, problem solving, decision making, comprehension, and production of

language); changes in mood and behavior (depression, impulsivity, aggression, anger, irritability, and even self-injurious or suicidal behavior); and dementia. Initial signs and symptoms do not typically appear until decades after the head trauma has occurred (i.e. ages 40-50).

4) Chronic Traumatic Encephalomyopathy (CTEM) – a small percentage of individuals with CTE may develop this progressive motor neuron disease with symptoms including significant weakness, atrophy (muscle wasting), spasticity (muscle stiffness), and fasciculations (uncontrolled twitching of muscle).

Assessment of Concussions

Assessment of a concussion involves a neurological examination (i.e. testing vision, hearing, sensation, muscle strength, balance, coordination, and reflexes) and neuropsychological tests measuring cognitive and other mental functioning (e.g. intelligence, problem solving, memory, concentration, attention, impulse control, and reaction time).

Brain imaging can be effective in determining structural abnormalities in the brain following a traumatic injury. Imaging studies can reveal skull fractures, internal bleeding, and brain lesions. Imaging tests such as a computerized tomography (CT) scan and magnetic resonance imaging (MRI) may be used to view bleeding in the brain or to diagnose complications that may occur after a concussion. Observation (hospitalization) may be required depending on the extent of injury and risk for complications.

Management of Concussion

Management of a concussion involves rest and avoiding general physical exertion or any vigorous activities. Rest may also include limiting activities that require thinking and mental concentration such as playing video games, watching TV, and schoolwork. Pain medication may be recommended for headaches.

Interviewing, symptom checklists, computerized neuropsychological testing, and other tests (e.g. vestibular balance testing) are used to evaluate cognitive and neurobehavioral improvement. Regarding athletes, baseline testing is performed preseason and used comparatively in evaluating the extent of symptoms and impairment when injury occurs. The comparative testing plays a role in indicating when it is safe to return an athlete to play.

IV. BRAIN HEALTH MAINTENANCE

1) **THE EFFECTS OF EXERCISE ON THE BRAIN**

Long-term vs short-term effects of exercise

Consistent aerobic exercise has been associated with long-term positive effects on the brain including improvements in executive functions (e.g. reasoning, problem-solving, cognitive flexibility) and aspects of memory. These effects have had significant implications for improving academic performance in children and college students, preserving cognitive function in older individuals, improving productivity in adults, preventing or treating certain neurological disorders, and improving overall quality of life. Increased nerve cell growth, increased nerve cell plasticity (i.e. capacity for nerve cell to adapt to stimuli), and increased signaling among nerve cells and other brain chemicals (e.g. hormones, growth factor) are some of the neurobiological factors believed to underlie the long-term effects of exercise.

The "runner's high" (or "rower's high") is a short-term euphoria or sense of elation that occurs after a sustained period of exercise and, according to some researchers, has been associated with the release of brain chemicals including phenethylamine (a stimulant), β-endorphin (an opioid), and anandamide (a cannabinoid).

Exercise and mental conditions

Addiction

Consistent aerobic exercise (e.g. endurance exercise such as marathon running) has been associated with preventing the development of certain drug addictions and with working as an adjunct treatment particularly for stimulant addiction.

Attention deficit hyperactivity disorder

When combined with stimulant medication (e.g. Adderall, Ritalin), regular aerobic exercise is an effective treatment for ADHD in children and adults. The effects of regular aerobic exercise include improved motor and cognitive function (i.e. attention, inhibitory control, and planning, faster information processing speed, and better memory); better self-esteem; decreased anxiety and depression; better academic performance; and improved social behavior.

Major depression

Physical exercise has been associated with a significant and persistent antidepressant effect and an improved overall quality of life. Exercise has been used as a treatment in conjunction with antidepressant medication for depression. In addition, yoga may be effective in alleviating symptoms of prenatal depression.

Other

Physical exercise is associated with a lower incidence of dementia, a reduced rate of cognitive decline, and an improved ability to perform activities of daily living in individuals with Alzheimer's disease. In addition, improvements in cognitive function have been observed in individuals with Parkinson's disease who engaged in regular exercise.

2) SLEEP

The stages of sleep may be divided into non-Rapid Eye Movement (non-REM) sleep and Rapid Eye Movement (REM) sleep. Most of the evening is spent in non-REM sleep (approximately 80%) with REM sleep comprising approximately 20% of the night. The activity occurring during each stage is outlined below.

<u>Stages of Sleep</u>
1) Non-REM (non-rapid eye movement) sleep:
a) Stage I - light, transitional, falling into sleep.
b) Stage II - onset of moderate, "true" sleep (occurs within 15-20 minutes); more than 50% of the night is spent in this phase which has been associated with the regulation of hormones that affect stress, appetite, biological rhythms, cell growth, and cell healing.
c) Stage III— occurs within 45 minutes of stages I & II; deep phase of sleep associated with growth, building, and repair of cells.
d) Stage IV— deep sleep continues; associated with growth, building, and repair of cells.

2) Rapid Eye Movement (REM) sleep: 1st REM period occurs approximately 45 minutes after Stage IV; periods get progressively longer through the night (stages III & IV become shorter); sleep becomes lighter and dreaming occurs; skeletal muscle tone is inhibited; and body temperature is decreased.

Insomnia

Insomnia has been described as a persistent difficulty falling or staying asleep, accompanied by an impairment in daytime function. It is a common condition affecting approximately one in three adults in the U.S. Severe, persistent insomnia adversely affecting function is associated with increased risk of depression, substance use, and medical problems.

Risk Factors For Impaired Sleep in the Sport Environment

1. Scheduling - regular sleep patterns can be disrupted by the timing of practices, travel, and competition.

2. Intense exercise in the evening can interfere with regular sleep patterns.

3. For students, the time demand of both athletics and academics can interfere as well.

4. Social events that compromise sleep—sleep after a practice or game plays a role in the brain's consolidating experience from the day's activities and aids in repairing the body.

Effect of Inadequate Sleep on Athletic Performance:

1. Decreased reaction time.

2. Decreased cognitive function, potentially limiting one's capacity to learn or remember plays or instructions.

3. Hormonal abnormalities (e.g. decreased testosterone).

4. Changes in metabolism which may lead to changes in appetite and overeating.

5. Decreased capacity to regulate emotions.

<u>Interventions</u>

Disrupted sleep may be re-regulated through sleep hygiene (i.e. measures to facilitate a normal sleep pattern without using medications) or, in severe cases, through the limited use of medications.

Sleep Hygiene—Example

1) Begin an unwinding routine at least 1hr before bedtime. During this time wind down stimulating or disruptive influences (e.g. video games, internet or tv channel surfing, stressful interactions with others).

2) Set a regular bedtime and make efforts to adhere to it even if not tired.

3) Make efforts to arise at the same time each morning.

4) Practice relaxation exercises in the evening (e.g. breathing, progressive muscle relaxation—See pages 12-16 of this guide).

5) Ensure a comfortable sleep space.

6) Limit activating substances (e.g. caffeine, alcohol, nicotine) especially in the later part of the day.

7) Get support for any psychological issues, if they are contributing factors to a sleep disturbance.

Coaches, trainers, and administrators should pay close attention to how scheduled activities influence their athletes' patterns of and opportunities for sleep and consider revising team schedules if necessary. Screening and communicating with athletes about the importance of adequate sleep for optimal athletics performance may help individuals prevent untoward sleep disturbances.

3) NUTRITION FOR OPTIMAL BRAIN & NEUROMUSCULAR FUNCTION

The nervous system is a complex network of neural cells that transmit messages to and from the brain and spinal cord to various parts of the body.   The system may be divided into the central and peripheral nervous systems. The central nervous system is made up of the brain and spinal cord and the peripheral nervous system is comprised of the somatic and autonomic nervous systems. The somatic nervous system consists of a) sensory fibers that carry information from the periphery of the body to the spinal cord and brain and b) motor fibers that carry central impulses to the periphery to stimulate skeletal muscle. The autonomic system consisting of sympathetic, parasympathetic, and other nerves fibers, control involuntary functions of the body such as heartbeat and digestion. Optimal function of the nervous system is vital for athletic performance. In this section, key nutrients providing nourishment to cells of the system are outlined.

Nutrients

Nutrients required for survival can be divided into two categories: macronutrients and micronutrients. Macronutrients are nutrients required in large ("macro") amounts and micronutrients are those required in small ("micro") amounts. Macronutrients include carbohydrate, fat, water, and protein. Micronutrients include vitamins, minerals (such as copper, iron, selenium, and zinc), and phytochemicals. Minerals such as calcium, sodium, magnesium, potassium, phosphorus, and sulfur are sometimes known as macronutrients (or "macro-minerals") because they are necessary in large quantities compared to other vitamins and minerals.

Macronutrients & Macro-minerals

Macronutrients

Carbohydrates (glucose). The body breaks down carbohydrate to form glucose, the main source of energy for the body's cells. The brain uses a tremendous amount of the body's glucose to fuel its cells (i.e. the brain is only 3% of the body's weight but consumes more than 25% of the body's glucose for fuel). Glucose is not capable of being stored in the brain cells so must constantly be supplied to the brain. Therefore, a steady, regular balance of carbohydrates is important for fueling the brain. Carbohydrate intake is associated with decreased levels of ammonia which can be toxic to the brain and impair metabolic processes in muscle. Deficits in glucose are associated with sluggishness, dizziness, and confusion. Healthy sources of carbohydrate include oats, lentils, figs, sweet potatoes, and rice bran.

Fats (omega-3 & omega-6 fatty acids). Omega fatty acids are essential building blocks for the brain cell membrane or wall and function to help brain cells communicate via neurotransmitters (i.e. brain chemicals that mediate communication between brain cells). They may also play a role in reducing inflammation in the brain. Deficiency in omega fatty acids has been associated with impaired memory and mental conditions including depression and ADHD. Foods rich in omega fatty acids include salmon, sardines, flaxseed, walnuts, sesame seeds, pumpkin seeds, peanuts, and soybeans.

Water. Our bodies are comprised of approximately 66% water. The brain consists of about 75% water (bones consist of about 22%; muscles around 75% , and blood approximately 92%). Water plays a significant role in functions including carrying nutrients and oxygen to all cells in the body; absorbing nutrients and converting food into energy; removing waste; moistening oxygen for breathing; regulating body temperature; protecting and cushioning vital organs; and cushioning joints.

Protein. Next to water, protein makes up most of the weight of our bodies. Muscles, organs, hair, nails, and ligaments are all composed of protein. In addition, the hormones and enzymes that cause chemical changes and control all body processes are made of proteins. Brain cells communicate with one another via chemical messengers (i.e. neurotransmitters) which are usually made of amino acids, the building blocks of protein. Poultry, seafood, and lean meat are the richest sources, as are dairy products, legumes, nuts, and seeds.

Macro-minerals

Calcium. Calcium is important for muscle contraction and energy metabolism. Sources include yogurt, cheese, almonds, sardines, sesame seeds.

Sodium. Sodium regulates the total amount of water in the body and is vital for the conduction of nerve impulses by brain cells. Sodium imbalance is associated with confusion and severe imbalances can be serious and life-threatening (e.g. potentially causing a seizure). Healthy foods high in sodium include beets and celery.

Magnesium. Magnesium assists in metabolizing glucose for energy and plays a role in muscle contraction. Sources include green leafy vegetables, garlic, seeds, nuts, and bran.

Potassium. Potassium is an element that is essential for keeping a normal water balance between the cells and body fluids. It also plays a key role in the response of nerves to stimulation and in the contraction of muscles. Foods high in potassium include bananas, cantaloupe, grapefruit, oranges, tomato or prune juice, honeydew melon, prunes, molasses, and potatoes.

Phosphorus. The main function of phosphorus is in the formation of bones and teeth. However, it also plays an important role in how the body uses carbohydrates and fats and makes protein for the growth, maintenance, and repair of cells and tissues. Phosphorus helps the body make adenosine triphosphate (ATP), a molecule the body uses to store energy. It also assists in kidney function, muscle contractions, normal heartbeat, and nerve signaling. Sources include meat, milk, and whole grain breads.

Sulfur. Sulfur is a component of four amino acids: methionine, cysteine, cystine, and taurine. Sulfur performs a number of important functions such as providing a place for these amino acids to bond together, thus solidifying a protein structure. Foods rich in sulfur include eggs, legumes, whole grains, garlic, onions, brussel sprouts, and cabbage.

Micronutrients

Vitamins

Vitamin B6. Vitamin B6 helps the body to make antibodies (i.e. proteins that help fight diseases), to maintain normal nerve function, and to make hemoglobin (which carries oxygen in the red blood cells to the tissues). It also breaks down proteins and keeps blood sugar (glucose) in normal ranges. B6 deficiency is not common in the US, but may result in confusion, mood instability, and dysfunction of peripheral nerves (i.e. peripheral neuropathy). Vitamin B6 is found in the highest quantities in potatoes, bananas, chick peas, and oatmeal.

Vitamin B7 (Biotin, also known as vitamin H). Biotin plays an important role in converting carbohydrates, fats, and proteins into energy. Sources include peanut butter, oats, egg yolks, hazelnuts, and almonds.

Vitamin B9 (folate, folic acid). As with other B vitamins, folic acid helps the body convert food (carbohydrates) into fuel (glucose) which is used to produce energy for brain cells. It also helps the body produce its genetic material (DNA and RNA) and use fats and protein. It works closely with vitamin B12 to produce red blood cells and to help iron function properly in the body. It works with vitamins B6, B12, and other nutrients to control blood levels of the amino acid homocysteine which, in high levels, can impair function of brain cells.

Folate deficiency has been associated with cognitive problems and increased risk for depression. Folate is found in leafy greens, citrus fruits, peas, and beans.

Vitamin B12. Vitamin B12 plays a part in forming red blood cells and converting food into energy. It also ensures that the brain and muscles communicate efficiently which affects muscle growth and coordination. B12 comes almost solely from animal products like meat (especially liver), seafood, eggs, milk, and cheese, so it may be necessary for strict vegetarians and vegans to supplement.

Vitamin C. Vitamin C is a powerful antioxidant that aids in metabolizing carbohydrates for fuel, helps the body absorb iron, and protects the body from infection and exercise-induced oxidative stress. Best sources include green peppers, broccoli, blackcurrants, and citrus fruits.

Vitamin D. Vitamin D influences certain proteins that aid in neuron growth and development. It takes part in many other important aspects of brain function including synaptic plasticity, learning, memory, the activity of neurotransmitters, and certain motor processes. Vitamin D helps the body absorb calcium and phosphorus. Calcium is essential for muscle contractions, while phosphorus is involved in the synthesis of adenosine triphosphate (ATP), the useable form of energy in the body. Long-term vitamin D deficiency in humans (i.e. several years) has been associated with cognitive and mood disorders. Sources of vitamin D include oily fish, olive oil, eggs, yoghurt, and sunflower seeds.

Vitamin E. Vitamin E has antioxidant properties and helps cell membrane recovery from oxidative stress, such as from exercise. Sources include nuts and seeds.

Minerals

Copper. Copper is the third most abundant trace mineral in the body. Copper enzymes regulate various cell functions such as energy production, iron metabolism, connective tissue maturation, and neurotransmission. It is associated with protecting the cardiovascular, nervous, and skeletal systems (it is a factor in strengthening tendons). Sources include peanuts, sardines, crab, and sunflower seeds.

Iron. Iron forms part of hemoglobin, the component of red blood cells that attaches oxygen and transports it from the lungs to all tissues of the body. It is essential for maintaining high energy levels and it plays a role in keeping the immune system functioning optimally. Sources include dried apricots, sardines, bran cereals, and venison.

Selenium. Selenium is associated with preventing depression and impeding free radical damage from exercise. Food sources include fresh tuna, sunflower seeds, whole-meal bread, and brazil nuts.

Zinc. Zinc enables the body to produce muscle-building testosterone. It also promotes recovery from exercise, boosts fertility, and increases the number of immune cells that fight infection.   Food sources include red meat, eggs, pulses, pumpkin seeds, and cheese.

Phytochemicals

Phytochemicals are chemical compounds derived from plant sources. There are a number of types of phytochemicals and one of the most significant groups is the *flavonoids*. Flavonoids increase levels of antioxidants and anti-inflammatory compounds that play a role in decreasing damage to brain cells. Flavonoids boost the brain's ability to form new neurons; prevent brain cells from dying; and enhance "synaptic plasticity," the ability of neurons to form and reform connections with one another. These processes, particularly synaptic plasticity, are considered to be the bases for learning, memory, and cognition in general. Flavonoids are found in plant-derived foods such as blueberries, apples, citrus fruits, black tea, green tea, cocoa, beer, and wine.

V. OVERVIEW OF BANNED SUBSTANCES AFFECTING ATHLETIC PERFORMANCE

Performance enhancing drugs (PEDs) have been described as substances that have the potential to improve physical or mental performance in humans. The term "ergogenic" refers to those drugs or aids that enhance physical or athletic performance while drugs improving cognitive or mental functions are referred to as "nooptropic." Athletic associations and leagues governing the activities and conduct of collegiate, Olympic/Paralympic, and professional athletes have adopted specific policies regarding the use and abuse of substances that are illegal or performance-enhancing. While policies of each governing body vary, they generally include guidance on specific banned substances, drug testing procedures for prohibited substances, disciplinary action for violations, and resources for treatment.

Categorization of PEDs has varied among sources but classes of drugs commonly banned by anti-doping agencies, associations, and leagues include illicit or illegal substances; steroids; hormones; diuretics or masking agents; stimulants; anti-estrogen drugs; beta blockers; and beta-2 agonists. Many of these substances have psychoactive effects or the ability to alter thoughts, emotions, and behavior (e.g. stimulants, steroids, hormones, alcohol, beta-blockers, and several illicit street drugs). Caffeine is a substance that has been on the border, considered a performance enhancer by some but not others.

Illegal Substances. In the US, illegal substances commonly banned include narcotics (e.g. heroin and other illegal opiates), illicit street drugs (e.g. cocaine, crystal meth, mushrooms), and, in several states, cannabis. Psychological effects of stimulants (e.g. cocaine, methamphetamine) and cannabis can be found on pages 88-92 of this guide. The psychological effects of opiates include euphoria and psychosis (e.g. paranoia, hallucinations). Irritability, depression, cravings, and anxiety have been associated with opiate withdrawal. Hallucinogens such as mushrooms alter perception and may cause anxiety, mood swings, and psychosis.

Steroids. Drugs commonly known as steroids can be classified as anabolic (anabolic-androgenic) steroids or corticosteroids. Corticosteroids, such as cortisone or prednisone are often prescribed by medical doctors to control inflammation in the body. Corticosteroids are not the same as the anabolic steroids that are often linked with illegal use in sports. Anabolic steroids are synthetic versions of the male hormone testosterone which aid the body in building skeletal muscle.

They also delay fatigue and may create a feeling of euphoria. Other psychiatric effects associated with steroids include irritability, agitation, mania, and psychosis (e.g. delusions, hallucinations). Withdrawal symptoms can occur when steroids are stopped following regular use and include irritability, depression, fatigue, restlessness, loss of appetite, insomnia, reduced sex drive, and steroid cravings.

Peptide Hormones & Analogues. Human growth hormone (HGH) is a factor in promoting the growth of bone and muscle and in reducing fat. A synthetic injectable form of HGH has been abused, as it has been considered to speed healing from injuries, build lean muscle mass, reduce fat, and promote vitality. Psychological effects associated with HGH include depression and psychosis (paranoia, hallucinations, irrational/illogical thought).

Diuretics/Masking Agents. In sports, a masking agent is used to hide or prevent detection of a banned substance or illegal drug like anabolic steroids or stimulants. Diuretics ("water pills") are the simplest form of a masking agent and work by enhancing water loss, resulting in diluting the urine. Banned substances are more difficult to detect in diluted urine. Mood disturbance and confusion are adverse psychological side effects associated with diuretics.

Stimulants. Substances referred to as stimulants (e.g. ADHD medication such as Adderall, cocaine, methamphetamine) cause the release of excitatory neurochemicals in the brain, such as dopamine, to stimulate the central nervous system (CNS). They can induce heightened feelings of power, strength, self-assertion, and enhanced motivation. In addition, they have been associated with delaying the onset of fatigue, increasing alertness, and decreasing appetite. Other psychological effects of stimulants may be found on pages 91-92 of this guide.

Anti-Estrogen Drugs. There is evidence that anti-estrogen drugs increase the production of testosterone and can mask the use of some steroids. Psychological side effects associated with anti-estrogen drugs include insomnia, depression, anxiety, lethargy, and mood swings.

Beta-Blockers & Alcohol. Beta blockers are drugs prescribed by doctors commonly for high blood pressure and also for anxiety. They decrease heart rate, blood pressure, and tremulousness associated with anxiety.

They may be an advantage to athletes in sports such as rifle shooting or archery where nervousness and tremulous fine muscle movement can harm performance. Alcohol, a substance which may also calm nerves, is usually banned during competition and may be banned both inside and outside of competition for sports such as shooting and archery. Additional psychological effects of alcohol may be found on pages 84-87 of this guide. Adverse psychological side effects of beta blockers include sleep disturbance and depression.

Beta 2 Agonists. An agonist is a drug that stimulates natural processes in the body. A beta-2 agonist stimulates beta-2 cell receptors which are associated with opening bronchial airways, permitting more oxygen into the lungs. They are commonly prescribed by medical doctors for patients with asthma. In large doses, beta-2 agonists may act also as an anabolic agent (promoting weight gain in the form of muscle); reduce body fat percentage; and accelerate recovery rates. Anxiety is a psychological side effect which has been associated with beta-2 agonists.

Dietary supplements. While not banned substances, dietary supplements (including vitamins & minerals) are a risk. Supplements have not been well regulated and have the potential to cause positive drug test results. According to the United States Anti-Doping Agency

(USADA) that offers information regarding "risky" supplements, there have been commercially-sold dietary supplements that contain, for example, designer steroids, stimulants, diuretics, and hormone products.

Drug testing for illegal or performance-enhancing substances usually involves sampling body fluids such as blood and urine. Disciplinary action for violations varies among leagues but has included warnings, fines, suspensions, and dismissal. Athletes with substance use disorders are offered resources for treatment including detoxification and outpatient or inpatient drug rehabilitation programs.

Banned Substances Lists

Examples of banned substances for the National Collegiate Athletic Association (NCAA), which governs substance policy for college athletes in the United States, are highlighted in this section. The list is reviewed and updated annually and the current, official list may be found at ncaa.org.

The World Anti-Doping-Agency (WADA) has established standards for athletes competing worldwide (The World Anti-Doping Code) and their current list of banned substances may be found at wada-ama.org. The U.S. Anti-Doping Agency (USADA) is the national anti-doping organization (NADO) in the United States for Olympic, Paralympic, Pan American, and Parapan American sport. The USADA recognizes the same standards and list of prohibited substances as WADA.

Current substance use and anti-doping policies for professional organizations such as the National Football League (NFL), Major League Baseball (MLB), National Basketball Association (NBA), and National Hockey League (NHL) may be found through an online search (e.g. "NFL Banned Substances," etc) or by contacting their respective corporate offices (e.g. search online, "NFL Corporate Office", "MLB Corporate Office," etc).

NCAA Banned Drugs

The NCAA Bans the Following Classes of Drugs:

1. Alcohol and Beta Blockers (banned for rifle only).

2. Anabolic Agents.

3. Anti-estrogens.

4. Beta-2 Agonists.

5. Diuretics and Other Masking Agents.

6. Peptide Hormones and Analogues.

7. Stimulants.

8. Street Drugs.

9. *Any substance chemically related to these classes is also banned.

Drugs and Procedures Subject to Restrictions: beta-2 Agonists (permitted only by prescription and inhalation); blood doping; gene doping; local anesthetics (under some conditions); and manipulation of urine samples.

NCAA Nutritional/Dietary Supplements Warning:

"Before consuming any nutritional/dietary supplement product, review the product with the appropriate or designated athletics department staff. There are no NCAA approved supplement products. Dietary supplements, including vitamins and minerals, are not well regulated and may cause a positive drug test result. Student-athletes have tested positive and lost their eligibility from using dietary supplements. Many dietary supplements are contaminated with banned drugs not listed on the label. Any product containing a dietary supplement ingredient is taken at the athletes own risk and athletes are urged to check with their athletics department staff prior to using a supplement."

Examples of NCAA Banned Substances in Each Drug Class

The NCAA warns that no complete list of banned substances exists and that student-athletes should not rely on this list to rule out any label ingredient.

1. Alcohol and Beta Blockers (banned for rifle only): Alcohol; atenolol; metoprolol; nadolol; pindolol; propranolol; timolol.

2. Anabolic Agents (sometimes listed as a chemical formula, such as 3,6,17-androstenetrione): Androstenedione; boldenone; clenbuterol; DHEA (7-

Keto); epi-trenbolone; etiocholanolone; methasterone; methandienone; nandrolone; norandrostenedione; ostarine, stanozolol; stenbolone; testosterone; trenbolone; SARMS (ostarine).

3. Anti-Estrogens: Anastrozole; tamoxifen; formestane; ATD; clomiphene; SERMS (nolvadex); Arimidex; clomid; evista; fulvestrant; aromatase inhibitors (Androst-3, 5-dien-7, 17-dione).

4. Beta-2 Agonists: Bambuterol; formoterol; salbutamol; salmeterol; higenamine; norcoclaurine.

5. Diuretics (water pills) and Other Masking Agents: Bumetanide; chlorothiazide; furosemide; hydrochlorothiazide; probenecid; spironolactone (canrenone); triameterene; trichlormethiazide.

6. Peptide Hormones and Analogues: Growth hormone (HGH); human chorionic gonadotropin (hCG); erythropoietin (EPO); IGF-1.

7. Stimulants: Amphetamine (Adderall); caffeine (guarana); cocaine; ephedrine; methamphetamine (DMAA); methylphenidate (Ritalin); synephrine (bitter orange); methylhexaneamine, "bath salts" (mephedrone); octopamne; DMBA; phenethylamines (PEAs). Exceptions: phenylephrine and pseudoephedrine are not banned.

8. Street Drugs: Heroin; marijuana; tetrahydrocannabinol (THC); synthetic cannabinoids (e.g., spice, K2, JWH-018, JWH-073).

Additional examples of banned drugs can be found at:

 www.ncaa.org/drugtesting

Substances that are chemically related to any of the classes listed are also banned and it is the athlete's responsibility to check with his or her athletics department before using any substance.

The Resource Exchange Center (REC) provides information about ingredients in medications and nutritional/dietary supplements and can be contacted at 877-202-0769 or www.drugfreesport.com/rec password: ncaa1, ncaa2 or ncaa3.

VI. ATHLETES WITH DISABILITIES

Adapted sport is a means for individuals with disabilities to develop and maintain physical and psychological functioning, a healthy lifestyle, and a satisfying quality of life. The Americans with Disabilities Act of 1990 (ADA) requires that individuals with disabilities be given equal opportunity in employment, transportation, public accommodation, communications, and governmental activities. Academic institutions (both public and private) are public accommodations and, those offering sports programs, are obligated to provide reasonable accommodations for athletes with disabilities.

In an inclusive environment, both individuals with and without disabilities benefit. Students with disabilities in inclusive settings demonstrate improvements in standardized tests scores, social and communication skills, interaction with peers, and preparedness for life following graduation. In addition, their peers without disabilities tend to be positively affected and display enhanced self-esteem; a greater acceptance and valuing of individual differences; a genuine capacity for friendship; and an acquisition of new skills.

<u>Guidance for coaches working with athletes with disabilities</u>

Outlined below are a few ways that athletes with disabilities may be included in team activities:

1. Embrace the opportunity. A coach demonstrating acceptance results in team members being positive and accepting as well.

2. Focus on the individual as an athlete instead of focusing on the disability. The athlete wants to participate in sports for the same reasons as athletes without disabilities. Take time to sit down with the athlete to determine goals for participation and to outline strategies for achieving the goals. Also, have realistic but challenging expectations for the athlete, just as a coach would for other athletes on the team.

 3. Allow opportunities to be a leader. Allow the athlete to choose drills or lead a pep talk demonstrating a capacity to take charge.

4. Promote independence. If other athletes on the team are expected to complete certain tasks or chores, the athlete should be expected to follow the same rules. The athlete is allowed accommodations such as taking additional time or using a creative way to complete the task, but he or she must take responsibility for managing the task.

5. Work with the athlete to modify sport techniques. Be aware of the accommodations established by the sport's governing body and work with the athlete to find creative and effective ways to execute skills with success.

6. Be open to and seek advice. Talk with others who have experience working with athletes with disabilities. A good resource for information and support includes the National Center on Physical Activity and Disability (ncpad.org).

VII. REFERENCES

Mental Skills Training

Carlstedt, R. (2013). Evidence-Based Applied Sport Psychology: A Practitioner's Manual. New York, NY: Springer Publishing Company, LLC.

Cox, R. (2007). Sport Psychology: Concepts and Applications. New York: McGraw-Hill.

Davis, M, Eshelman, E, McKay, M. (2008). The Relaxation and Stress Reduction Workbook. Oakland, CA: New Harbinger Publications, Inc.

Hays, K (2009). Performance Psychology in Action: A Casebook for Working with Athletes, Performing Artists, Business Leaders, and Professionals in High-Risk Occupations. Washington, DC: American Psychological Association.

Jeste, D and Palmer, B (2015). Positive Psychiatry: A Clinical Handbook. Arlington, VA: American Psychiatric Publishing.

Mack, G and Casstevens, D (2001). Mind Gym: An athlete's Guide to Inner Excellence. New York, NY: McGraw-Hill.

Maxwell, J., Masters, R., and Poolton (2006). Performance breakdown in Sport: The roles of reinvestment and verbal knowledge. Research

Quarterly for Exercise and Sport, 77(2), 271-276.

McDuff, D (2012). Sports Psychiatry: Strategies for Life Balance and Peak Performance. Arlington, VA: American Psychiatric Publishing.

Murphy, S (2005). The Sport Psych Handbook. Champaign, IL: Human Kinetics Publishers, Inc.

Poolton, J., Masters, R., and Maxwell, J. (2005). The relationship between errorless learning conditions and subsequent performance. Human Movement Science, 24, 362-378.

Poolton, J., Maxwell, J., Masters, R., & Raab, M. (2006). Benefits of an external focus of attention: Common coding or conscious processing? Journal of Sport Sciences, 24(1), 89-99.

Sorenson, Lacey, et al. (2008). Listen up! The experience of music in sport - a phenomenological investigation. Athletic Insight: The Online Journal of Sport Psychology 2008 Vol.10 No.2, unpaginated. Retrieved from http://www.athleticinsight.com/Vol10Iss2/Music.htm.

General Mental Health

Adamson SJ, Kay-Lambkin FJ, Baker AL et al. (2010). An improved brief measure of cannabis misuse: the Cannabis Use Disorders Identification Test-Revised (CUDIT-R). Drug Alc Dep, 110:37-143.

American College of Sports Medicine. (2007). The Female Athlete Triad. Medicine and Science in Sports and Exercise, 39:10: 1-10.

American College of Sports Medicine, et al (2006). Psychological Issues Related to Injury in Athletes and the Team Physician: A Consensus Statement. Medicine & Science in Sports & Exercise, pp 2030-2034. DOI: 10.1249/MSS.0b013e31802b37a6

Bacon, V., & Russell, P. (2004). Addiction and the college athlete: The Multiple Addictive Behaviors Questionnaire (MABQ) with college athletes. The Sport Journal, 7(2).

Brown GT, Hainline B, Kroshus E, Wilfert M. (2014). Mind, Body and Sport: Understanding and Supporting Student-Athlete Mental Wellness. Retrieved from ncaa.org.

Buchanan, J. L. (2012). Prevention of depression in the college student population: A review of the literature. Archives of Psychiatric Nursing, 26(1), 21–42. doi:10.1016/j.apnu.2011.03.003. Retrieved from http://www.sciencedirect.com/science/article/pii

/S0883941711000379

Brooks MA, et al. (2016). Concussion Increases Odds of Sustaining a Lower Extremity Musculoskeletal Injury After Return to Play Among Collegiate Athletes. Am J Sports Med, 44(3):742-7. doi: 10.1177/0363546515622387.

Center for Behavioral Health Statistics and Quality (CBHSQ). (2015). Behavioral Health Trends in the United States: Results from the 2014 National Survey on Drug Use and Health. Rockville, MD: Substance Abuse and Mental Health Services Administration; 2015. HHS Publication No. SMA 15-4927, NSDUH Series H-50.

Danish, SJ, Forneris, T, Wallace, I. (2005). Sport-based life skills programming in the schools. School Sport Psychology: Perspectives, Programs, and Procedures, 21, 41- 62. doi: 10.1300/J008v21n02_04

Emmons RA, McCullough ME. (2003). Counting blessings versus burdens: an experimental investigation of gratitude and subjective well-being in daily life. J Pers Soc Psychol, 84(2):377-89.
Gilbert FC, et al. (2016). Association Between Concussion and Lower Extremity Injuries in Collegiate Athletes. Sports Health. pii: 1941738116666509.

Greenleaf C, Petrie, TA, Carter J et al. (2009). Female collegiate athletes: prevalence of eating disorders and disordered eating behaviors. J Am Coll Health, 57:489-

495.

Harmon KG, et al. (2013). American Medical Society for Sports Medicine position statement: concussion in sport. Br J Sports Med, 47(1):15-26. doi: 10.1136/bjsports-2012-091941.

Hill LS, Reid F, Morgan JF et al. (2010. SCOFF, the development of an eating disorder screening questionnaire. Int J Eat Disord, 43:344-351.

Leddy MH, Lambert MJ, Ogles BM. (1994). Psychological consequences of athletic injury among high-level competitors. Res Q Exerc Sport, 65:347-354.

Llewellyn T, et al. (2014). Concussion reporting rates at the conclusion of an intercollegiate athletic career. Clin J Sport Med, 24(1):76-9.

Lyubomirsky, S. (2008). The How of Happiness. New York, NY: Penguin Press.

Matheson GO. (2001). Maintaining professionalism in the athletic environment. Phys Sportsmed, 29(2).

Mathieu JE, Kukenberger MR, D'Innocenzo L, Reilly G. (2015). Modeling reciprocal team cohesion-performance relationships, as impacted by shared leadership and members' competence. J Appl Psychol, 100(3):713-34.

National Collegiate Athletic Association (NCAA). (2006). Division II model life skills resource. Retrieved from http://www.ncaa.org/sites/default/files/10_D2_LifeSkill s%2BDocument.pdf

NCAA Sport Science Institute and the NCAA. (2014). Inter-association consensus document: best practices for understanding and supporting student-athlete mental wellness. Retrieved from http://www.ncaa.org/sites/default/files/HS_Mental-Health-Best-Practices_20160317.pdf.

Neal TL, Diamond AB, Goldman S et al. (2013). Inter-association recommendations for developing a plan to recognize and refer student-athletes with psychological concerns at the collegiate level: an executive summary of a consensus statement. J Athl Train, 48:716-720.

NIH Institute on Alcohol Abuse and Alcoholism. (2016). Alcohol use disorder. Retrieved from https://www.niaaa.nih.gov/alcohol-health/overview-alcohol-consumption/alcohol-use-disorders

NIH Institute on Drug Abuse. (2014). Marijauna use and educational outcomes. Retrieved from https://www.drugabuse.gov/publications/finder/t/877/brain-and-addiction.NIH Institute on Drug Abuse. (2015). NIDA highlights drug use trends among college-age and young adults in new online resource. Retrieved from https://www.drugabuse.gov/news-events/news-releases/2015/05/nida-highlights-drug-use-trends-among-college-age-young-adults-in-new-online-resource.

NIH Institute on Drug Abuse. (2016). College and young adult drug use data now available online. Retrieved from https://www.drugabuse.gov/news-events/news-releases/2016/05/college-young-adult-drug-use-data-now-available-online.

Rauh MJ, Nichols JF, Barrack MT. (2010). Relationships among injury and disordered eating, menstrual dysfunction, and low bone mineral density in high school athletes: a prospective study. J Athl Train, 45:243-252.

Shirreffs SM, Maughan RJ. (2006). The effect of alcohol on athletic performance. Curr Sports Med Rep, 5:192-196.

Stein, C, Ackerman, K, Stracciolini, A. (2016). The Young Female Athlete (Contemporary Pediatric and Adolescent Sports Medicine). Switzerland: Springer International Publishing.

Sundgot-Borgen J. (1994). Risk and trigger factors for the development of eating disorders in female elite athletes. Med Sci Sports Exerc, 26:414-419.

Tartakovsky, M. (2016). Depression and Anxiety Among College Students. Psych Central. Retrieved on October 26, 2016, from http://psychcentral.com/lib/depression-and-anxiety-among-college-students/

Taylor J, Ogilvie B, Lavallee D. (2006). Career transition among athletes: is there life after sports? In Williams JM (ed) Applied sport psychology: Personal growth to peak performance (5th ed.). Boston, Mass: McGraw Hill.

Taylor J, Ogilvie B. (1994). A conceptual model of adaptation to retirement among athletes. J App Sport Psych, 6:1-20.

Thompson BM, et al. (2015). Team cohesiveness, team size and team performance in team-based learning teams. Med Educ, 49(4):379-85.

Tuckman J, Lorge I. (1953). Retirement and the Industrial Worker. New York, NY: Macmillan.

U.S. Department of Health and Human Services. (2012). Results from the 2012 National Survey on Drug Use and Health: Mental Health Findings. Rockville, MD: Substance Abuse and Mental Health Services Administration; NSDUH Series H-47, HHS Publication No. (SMA) 13-4805.

U.S. Department of Health and Human Services (HHS), Office of the Surgeon General. (2016). Facing Addiction in America: The Surgeon General's Report on Alcohol, Drugs, and Health. Washington, DC: HHS.

Wang F, et al. (2012).Long-term association between leisure-time physical activity and changes in happiness: analysis of the Prospective National Population Health Survey. Am J Epidemiol, 176(12):1095-100.

Wasserman EB, et al. Epidemiology of Sports-Related Concussions in National Collegiate Athletic Association Athletes From 2009-2010 to 2013-2014: Symptom Prevalence, Symptom Resolution Time, and Return-to-Play Time. Am J Sports Med, 44(1):226-33. doi: 10.1177/0363546515610537.

Weigand S, Cohen J, Merenstein D. (2013). Susceptibility for depression in current and retired student athletes. Sports Health 5:263-266.

Yang J, Cheng G, Zhag Y et al. (2014). Influence of symptoms of depression and anxiety on injury hazard among collegiate American football players. Res Sports Med, 22:147-160.

Yuso DA, Buckman JF, White HR et al. (2008). Risk for excessive alcohol use and drinking-related problems in college student athletes. Addict Behav, 33:1546-1556.

Brain Health

American College of Sports Medicine, American Dietetic Association, and Dietitians of Canada, Joint Position Stand. (2009). Nutrition and Athletic Performance. Medicine and Science in Sports and Exercise, 109:3:509-527.

American Dietetic Association; Dietitians of Canada; American College of Sports Medicine. (2009). American College of Sports Medicine position stand. Nutrition and athletic performance. Med Sci Sports Exerc, 41(3):709-31.

Benardot, D. (2011). Advanced Sports Nutrition-2nd Edition. Champaign, IL: Human Kinetics.

De Sousa EF, Da Costa TH, Nogueira JA, Vivaldi LJ. (2008). Assessment of nutrient and water intake among adolescents from sports federations in the Federal District, Brazil. Br J Nutr, 99(6):1275-83.

Digate Muth N. (2015). Sports Nutrition for Health Professionals. Philadelphia, PA. F.A. Davis Company.

Erickson KI, Hillman CH, Kramer AF (2015). "Physical activity, brain, and cognition". Current Opinion in Behavioral Sciences. 4: 27–32. doi:10.1016/j.cobeha.2015.01.005

Gomez-Pinilla F, Hillman C (2013). "The influence of exercise on cognitive abilities". Compr. Physiol. 3 (1):

403–428. doi:10.1002/cphy.c110063

Guiney H, Machado L (2013). "Benefits of regular aerobic exercise for executive functioning in healthy populations". Psychon Bull Rev. 20 (1): 73–86. doi:10.3758/s13423-012-0345-4

Lemola S, Ledermann T, Friedman EM. (2013). Variability of sleep duration is related to subjective sleep quality and subjective well-being: an actigraphy study. PLoS One, 8(8):e71292. doi: 10.1371/journal.pone.0071292.

Lund HG, Reider BD, Whiting AB et al. (2010). Sleep patterns and predictors of disturbed sleep in a large population of college students. J Adolesc Health, 46:124-132.

Mah CD, Mah KE, Kezirian EJ et al. (2011). The effects of sleep extension on the athletic performance of collegiate basketball players. Sleep, 34:943-950.

Parnell JA, Wiens KP, Erdman KA. (2016). Dietary Intakes and Supplement Use in Pre-Adolescent and Adolescent Canadian Athletes. Nutrients, 8(9). pii: E526. doi: 10.3390/nu8090526.

Pöchmüller M, Schwingshackl L, Colombani PC, Hoffmann G. (2016). A systematic review and meta-analysis of carbohydrate benefits associated with randomized controlled competition-based performance trials. J Int Soc Sports Nutr, 13:27. doi:

10.1186/s12970-016-0139-6.

Russell M, Benton D, Kingsley M. (2014). Carbohydrate ingestion before and during soccer match play and blood glucose and lactate concentrations. J Athl Train, 49(4):447-53.

Savis JC (1994). Sleep and athletic performance: overview and implications for sport psychology. Sport Psychologist, 8:111-125.

Schuch FB, et al. (2016). "Exercise improves physical and psychological quality of life in people with depression: A meta-analysis including the evaluation of control group response". Psychiatry Res. 241: 47–54. doi:10.1016/j.psychres.2016.04.054

Shriver LH, Bets NM, Wollenberg G, (2013). Dietary intakes and eating habits of college athletes: are female college athletes following current sports nutrition standards? J AM Coll Health, 61(1): 10-6.

Overview of Banned Substances

Buckman JF, Farris SG, Yusko DA. (2013). A national study of substance use behaviors among NCAA male athletes who use banned performance enhancing substances. Drug Alcohol Depend, 131(1-2):50-5. doi: 10.1016/j.drugalcdep.2013.04.023.

Momaya A, Fawal M, Estes R. (2015). Performance-enhancing substances in sports: a review of the literature. Sports Med, 45(4):517-31. doi: 10.1007/s40279-015-0308-9.

Morente-Sánchez J, Zabala M. (2013). Doping in sport: a review of elite athletes' attitudes, beliefs, and knowledge. Sports Med, 43(6):395-411. doi: 10.1007/s40279-013-0037-x.

National Collegiate Athletic Association (NCAA). (2016). 2016-17 Banned Drug List. Retrieved from http://www.ncaa.org/2016-17-ncaa-banned-drugs-list

U.S. Anti-doping Agency (USADA). (2014). Supplement 411: Realize, Recognize, Reduce. Retrieved from http://www.usada.org/substances/supplement-411/

World Anti-Doping Agency (WADA). (2016). WADA Ethics Panel: Guiding Values in Sport and Anti-Doping. Retrieved from https://www.wada-ama.org/en/resources/general-anti-doping-information/wada-ethics-panel-guiding-values-in-sport-and-anti-doping.

World Anti-Doping Agency (WADA). (2017). Prohibited
List. Retrieved from https://wada-main-
prod.s3.amazonaws.com/resources/files/2016-09-29_-
_wada_prohibited_list_2017_eng_final.pdf

Athletes with Disabilities

Adapted Swim Committee (2001). Including swimmers with a disability: A guide for coaches. Retrieved from http://www.usaswimming.org/USASWeb/_Rainbow/Documents/db2d2891-6891-4e56-b1c4-47d209afe9f8/adapted_coaches_brochure.pdf.

Americans With Disabilities Act of 1990, Pub. L. No. 101-336, 104 Stat. 328 (1990).

Hanrahan, S. (2015). Psychological Skills Training for Athletes With Disabilities. Australian Psychologist (50) pp 102–105. DOI: 10.1111/ap.12083

Power-deFur L, Orelove F. (1997). Inclusive Education: Practical Implementation of the Least Restrictive Environment. by Gaithersburg, MD: Aspen Publishers.

Shapiro, D, et al. (2016). Quality of life and psychological affect related to sport participation in children and youth athletes with physical disabilities: A parent and athlete perspective. Disability and Health Journal, 9(3), 385 – 391.

VIII. INDEX